VISUAL
FIELDS

VISUAL FIELDS

Neil Choplin, MD
Naval Medical Center
San Diego, CA

Russell Edwards, MD
Naval Medical Center
San Diego, CA

II\ The Basic Bookshelf for Eyecare Professionals

Series Editors: Janice K. Ledford • Ken Daniels • Robert Campbell

SLACK Incorporated, 6900 Grove Road, Thorofare, NJ 08086

Publisher: John H. Bond
Editorial Director: Amy E. Drummond
Creative Director: Linda Baker
Assistant Editor: Jennifer Stewart

Choplin, Neil T.
    Visual fields/Neil T. Choplin, Russell P. Edwards
        p. cm.
    Includes bibliographical references and index.
    ISBN 1-55642-363-2 (alk. paper)
    1. Perimetry.
    2. Visual Fields.
I. Edwards, Russell P. II. Title. III. Series.
RE79.P4C463 1998
617.7'5--dc21

                                                              97-48545
                                                                   CIP

Printed in the United States of America

Published by: SLACK Incorporated
               6900 Grove Road
               Thorofare, NJ 08086-9447 USA
               Telephone: 609-848-1000
               Fax: 609-853-5991
               World Wide Web: http://www.slackinc.com

Contact SLACK Incorporated for more information about other books in this field or about the availability of our books from distributors outside the United States.

Last digit is print number: 10 9 8 7 6 5 4 3 2 1

Dedication

This book is dedicated to everyone who is committed to the improvement of eyecare.

Contents

Acknowledgments

The authors gratefully acknowledge the guidance and patience of their editors, Jan Ledford and Amy Drummond. Geri Beuke of the American Optometric Association Paraoptometric Section and Marsha Price, OptT, chairman of the National Paraoptometric Registration Exam Committee, both assisted in helping us understand what optometric assistants and technicians need to know about visual fields.

About the Authors

Neil Choplin, MD is a graduate of New York University with a bachelor's degree in mathematics. He received his medical degree from New York Medical College, served a general surgery internship at Long Island Jewish Hillside Medical Center, and did a residency in ophthalmology at Nassau County Medical Center. Dr. Choplin entered military service after completing residency training and served 4 years at the Naval Hospital in Philadelphia. After completion of a glaucoma fellowship at the Wills Eye Hospital, Dr. Choplin transferred to the Naval Medical Center in San Diego, where he is currently the chairman of the Department of Ophthalmology, director of the glaucoma service, and president of the San Diego County Ophthalmological Society. He holds the rank of captain in the Navy Medical Corps and is certified by the American Board of Ophthalmology. Dr. Choplin has extensive experience in visual field testing and has written numerous related articles and textbook chapters. He has also authored a book on visual field testing with the Humphrey Field Analyzer. He serves as a commissioner on the Joint Commission for Allied Health Personnel in Ophthalmology™ (JCAHPO™), representing the Society of Military Ophthalmologists. San Diego has been particularly good to Dr. Choplin, his wife Lynn, and teenage daughters Danielle and Suzanne.

Russell Edwards, MD received his bachelor's degree in chemistry from the University of Missouri in Columbia ad his medical degree from the University of Alabama in Birmingham. He then entered the United States Navy and served his internship at the Regional Naval Medical Center in Portsmouth, Va. Following his ophthalmology residency training at the Naval Hospital in San Diego, Calif., Dr. Edwards served as a fellow in neuro-ophthalmology and orbital surgery at the Allegheny campus of the Medical College of Pennsylvania. A captain in the Navy Medical Corps, he is currently assigned to the Naval Medical Center in San Diego where he is the assistant chairman of the Department of Ophthalmology and the director of the neuro-ophthalmology and oculoplastics services. Dr. Edwards has authored a book on visual field testing and has been teaching visual field testing for many years. He lives in San Diego with his wife, Deborah, and his two sons, Zachary and Jeffrey.

Preface

The discipline of eyecare is concerned with the diagnosis and management of diseases affecting the entire visual system. Many disorders can be adequately detected by visual acuity testing or by direct examination of the eye with the slit lamp biomicroscope, the direct ophthalmoscope, or the indirect ophthalmoscope. Loss of visual function in many eye disorders is not limited to central vision and may not even affect visual acuity early in the course of the disease. Testing of the peripheral (side) vision, or the visual field, becomes important for the detection and monitoring of progression for such disorders. This book is about the visual field and how to examine it.

Visual field testing, also known as perimetry, is an art unto itself, and as such requires intensive instruction, patience, practice, and experience to master. The perimetrist must have knowledge of the visual pathways, the expected defects in the patient being tested, and the various techniques available to elicit them. In addition to knowledge and skill, the perimetrist must possess excellent interpersonal skills in order to help the patient perform to the best of his or her ability in what is often a difficult examination. A skilled perimetrist is a highly prized asset in the practice of an eyecare provider.

The majority of visual field test instruments today are computerized and automated. What this means is that the actual performance of the test (ie, presenting test objects to the patient), the recording of the patient's responses, the printing of the results, etc, are done by the machine itself. Why should a perimetrist need to know anything more than how to turn the machine on? Why would anyone need a book such as this one? The art of perimetry cannot be automated. All patients are different and respond to test situations differently. Patients must be prepared for the examination; they need to be instructed as to what to do and how to do it. The machine must be prepared for the patient—data must be entered, correcting lenses must be placed, and the patient must be positioned. Patients cannot be left alone while the test is being conducted. They need another human being nearby, someone with knowledge and skill, to help them perform properly. None of these activities can be computerized or left to a machine. Some eyecare practices still rely on manual techniques for visual field testing, and occasionally there are patients who cannot perform an automated test. The need still exists for knowledge of the available visual field test techniques and how to apply them in the appropriate clinical situation. However, it is not possible in a work of this size to cover every possible machine, manual or automated, on the market today nor those previously marketed. It is essential that the perimetrist thoroughly read the manual that comes with the instrument being used. The principles outlined in this book will apply to most test situations.

The authors are trained in the two main subspecialties in ophthalmology in which visual field testing is routine—glaucoma and neuro-ophthalmology. Between us we have about 22 years of experience with visual fields, mostly with the Humphrey Field Analyzer™ but also the with Amsler grid and the tangent screen. We have attempted to provide the reader with the benefit of our experiences; if a mistake is possible we probably have had to deal with it. We have devoted an entire section of the book to errors in visual field testing and how to minimize them. We hope that this information will prove useful. We understand that it is impossible to describe all possible test situations and talk about all types of machines, and undoubtedly there will be information missing that might be applicable in a particular practice setting. Please write to us in care of SLACK Incorporated and let us know what would be helpful to you.

The authors are active duty members of the United States Navy. We have no proprietary interest in any of the products described in this book. By discussion of a particular instrument, we intend no commercial endorsement of the product. The views and opinions expressed in this work are ours alone and are not intended to be construed as official opinions of the Department of the Navy, the Department of Defense, nor of the United States government.

Neil Choplin, MD

Introduction

Visual field testing has undergone "modernization" as equipment has changed to keep up with the times. Most perimetry is now computerized and automated. However, no machine can take the place of the perimetrist. A machine may be capable of performing some of the functions of the perimetrist, but it cannot fulfill the vital role played by the perimetrist in getting a patient through what is often a difficult examination. The role of visual field technician may have shifted from that of actually performing the examination to that of patient advocate and supporter, perhaps even a coach. As the reader goes through this book, the ever-present question should be, "What can I do to make this task easier, improve reliability, and present the best results possible to the eyecare professional who relies on the visual field information for proper diagnosis, follow-up, and care of the patient?"

In the material that follows, almost all techniques of perimetry will be discussed, and all have a place in modern eyecare. Most offices are equipped with automated perimeters. It is widely believed that not all patients can "survive" an examination on an automated perimeter. With proper support, education, periodic reinstruction, encouragement, periods of rest, and proper fine-tuning of technique, it is our belief that virtually all patients can be tested with automated perimetry. Therefore, the role of Goldmann perimetry has been somewhat downplayed in this text. Techniques such as static threshold testing on the Goldmann, for example, are best left to more complete texts on the subject. We have attempted to emphasize perimetric techniques that are common to all types of visual field testing situations, since common errors occur with all methods of testing.

The book begins with a description of what the visual field is and gives an overview of what visual field testing attempts to do. Terminology is discussed and common words are defined. The anatomy of the visual system is discussed with an emphasis on how lesions within the visual pathways give rise to the defects seen on perimetry. Next the various testing modalities are discussed, from simple screening techniques such as confrontation testing to a detailed description of automated perimetry. Emphasis is placed on visual field testing systems with explanations about how to organize and maintain efficient testing areas in a variety of clinical settings. An important chapter deals with common errors in visual field testing and offers tips on how to minimize them. We provide a small atlas of common visual field defects as determined mainly by automated perimetry using the Humphrey Field Analyzer™, representing a cross section of common disorders of the visual system.

We hope the material is interesting and useful. Perimetry occupies a large portion of our time, not only as clinicians but also as educators. We appreciate feedback from our readers and are always looking for tips on how to do things better. Feel free to pass suggestions along to us.

Neil Choplin, MD
Russell Edwards, MD

The Study Icons

The *Basic Bookshelf for Eyecare Professionals* is quality educational material designed for professionals in all branches of eyecare. Because so many of you want to expand your careers, we have made a special effort to include information needed for certification exams. When these study icons appear in the margin of a *Series* book, it is your cue that the material next to the icon (which may be a paragraph or an entire section) is listed as a criteria item for a certification examination. Please use this key to identify the appropriate icon:

OptA   optometric assistant

OptT   optometric technician

OphA   ophthalmic assistant

OphT   ophthalmic technician

OphMT   ophthalmic medical technologist

LV   low vision subspecialty

Srg   ophthalmic surgical assisting subspecialty

CL   contact lens registry

Optn   opticianry

RA   retinal angiographer

Section I

INTRODUCTION TO VISUAL FIELDS

Chapter 1

Basics of Visual Field Testing

KEY POINTS

- The visual field refers to that portion of visual space which is visible to an individual at any given moment.

- Perimetry is the science of measuring the peripheral vision in order to determine the visual field.

- The visual field has been likened to an "island of vision in a sea of blindness." Drawing a "map" of the island of vision is the goal of perimetry.

- Many aspects of perimetry may be performed by automated machines, but a skilled, knowledgeable technician is still required for optimal results.

Definition of the Visual Field

When we think of vision, we usually think of the sense that allows us to look at something with the ability to make out its details—size, shape, color, texture, etc. We rely most heavily on the portion of our visual system that is designed for perceiving fine detail—picking up a small object from the table, reading the newspaper, dialing the telephone, and so on. The portion of the visual system used for these tasks begins with the highly specialized area of the retina known as the macula, more specifically a small depression in the center of the macula (the fovea), which is no bigger than the head of a pin. This aspect of visual function is known as central vision because usually what we look at is in the center of our field of view and also because the center of the retina is the viewing screen. However, we are also wired for a much wider view and have the ability to see coarser detail to the side of the center. This side, or peripheral, vision serves a number of purposes. One is to give us an awareness of our surroundings, ie, a "visual context" for what we are looking at. Another purpose of our peripheral vision is to detect motion and alert us that something or someone has entered our environment or that the environment has changed. We may then use our eye, neck, and body muscles to move our eyes into a position that allows us to focus our central vision on the change in visual space. Our peripheral vision also helps us at night; the ratio of rods to cones is much higher outside of the macula, and thus the peripheral retina is more sensitive to low light levels. Of course, fine detail is not as sharp because the photoreceptors outside of the macula are not wired one-to-one with a retinal nerve fiber as are the cones within the fovea.

Even though peripheral vision is important, it would not be necessary to measure it if there were no diseases capable of affecting it. In fact, there are many diseases of the visual system that affect primarily the peripheral vision, at least early in the course of the disease. Glaucoma, for example, is a condition in which the nerve fibers that make up the optic nerve are gradually destroyed. The manner in which the fibers are destroyed is characteristic of the disease and affects only the peripheral vision until very late in the disease process. Because the central vision is affected late in the course of glaucoma, patients often have no symptoms to indicate that they have the disease. Glaucoma cannot be diagnosed strictly on the basis of intraocular pressure (IOP), however, because many people have pressures high enough to be considered "abnormal" yet may not actually have glaucoma. A measurement of the extent of the peripheral vision is thus essential to diagnose the disease.

The full extent of the peripheral vision is often referred to as the visual field. The visual field can be defined as that portion of space which is visible to an individual at any given moment. Although visual space is normally perceived with both eyes, for most purposes the visual field of each eye is measured separately. Once the field has been defined for each eye, the two visual fields can be compared to each other for asymmetry, compared to a "normal"' reference base for abnormality, and examined together to look for patterns suggestive of different conditions.

Perimetry is the science of measuring ("-metry") the peripheral ("peri-") vision in order to determine the visual field. Methods employed in perimetry have evolved and adapted to advances in technology, particularly electronics and computer science. Modern visual field testing as such is much more than a determination of the limits of visual space. Modern techniques allow for examination of the entire visual field, including the central field, and have helped to broaden our understanding of the conditions we are testing.

The Island of Vision

In 1930, Traquair likened the visual field of the eye to an "island of vision in a sea of blindness." This island (or hill) of vision analogy serves as the model for visual field testing (Figure 1-1). Perimetry is nothing more than determination of the dimensions of the island of vision, including its height and extent in all directions. It could be said that perimetry is simply a matter of drawing a map of the island of vision for the eye(s) being tested.

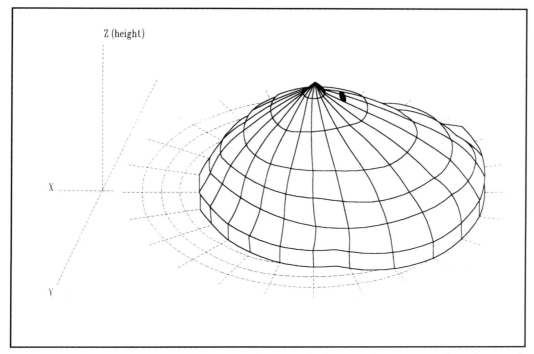

Figure 1-1. Three-dimensional representation of the island of vision. The positions along the X and Y axes represent points in the visual field centered around fixation, and the Z axis represents the height of the island (Drawing by Lynn R. Choplin).

Regardless of its extent or shape, an important aspect of the analogy is that the island of vision is a three-dimensional structure. For most "maps," the fovea is the visual field point where the X and Y coordinates correspond to (0,0). The location of the other visual field points can be expressed as an X,Y pair with respect to fixation. The unit used for the X and Y axes is degrees from fixation. The Z axis represents the height of the island of vision at the point (X,Y) and corresponds to the sensitivity of the retina at that point. The greater the sensitivity at any point, the greater the height of the island of vision. In the normal visual field the fovea is the "peak" of the island, since it has the greatest sensitivity. The normal extent of the island of vision is approximately 60° nasally (inward, or to the left in Figure 1-1), 60° superiorly (upward, or behind the peak and not visible in Figure 1-1), 70° to 75° inferiorly (downward in Figure 1-1), and 100° to 110° temporally (outward or to the right in Figure 1-1). The normal physiological blind spot, which corresponds to the location of the optic nerve head in the retina (it is a blind spot because the optic nerve head contains no photoreceptors) is centered slightly below the horizontal midline and 15.5° temporally (outward) relative to fixation. It measures approximately 5.5° wide and 7.5° high.

Mapping the Island of Vision

With the island of vision as an analogy for the visual field, perimetry becomes a matter of mapping the island. The method used to draw the map is not important as long as the map obtained is a true and accurate representation of the island for the eye being tested, and the information is presented in such a way as to be clinically useful. We have the problem of representing a three-dimensional structure (the island of vision) two-dimensionally, ie, on a piece of paper. The two ways this may be accomplished are depicted in Figure 1-2.

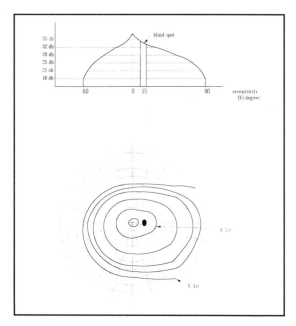

Figure 1-2. Vertical (top) and horizontal (bottom) "slices" through the island of vision. Vertical slices yield a profile of the island of vision along a given meridian, while horizontal slices yield a contour map (Adapted from Harrington DO. *The Visual Fields.* 4th ed. St Louis, Mo: CV Mosby; 1976. Drawing by Lynn R. Choplin).

Both methods involve drawing representative "slices" through the island of vision. The top of Figure 1-2 represents a vertical slice taken directly over the horizontal meridian and is drawn as it would appear if viewed head on. This is known as profile perimetry. The two dimensions represented are the horizontal extent along the chosen meridian and the height of the island of vision at the horizontal point. The height is determined by measuring the sensitivity of the retina at the test point. If multiple profiles were obtained along multiple meridia and then combined, a three-dimensional picture would be obtained.

The bottom of Figure 1-2 represents how the island of vision would appear if multiple horizontal cuts were obtained and stacked on top of each other. Each line represents the horizontal and vertical extent of the area of the visual field capable of seeing a stimulus of a given size and brightness. The view is directly over-head, looking down onto the surface of the island. The lines may be thought of as contour lines of the island of vision.

Visual Field Terminology

Perimetry

The dictionary defines *perimeter* as a "closed curve bounding a plane area," or the "outer limits of an area." It is derived from the Middle English, Latin, and Greek "peri" and "metron," meaning measure. Perimetry as applied to medicine is the art of defining the boundaries of the visual field and is interchangeable with visual field testing. The definition of the type of perimetry is based on the method used for the examination.

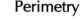

For the purposes of perimetry, the visual field is usually considered in two parts—the central visual field and the peripheral visual field. The terms are relevant to the naming of standard tests on some automated perimeters and may have slightly different meanings depending on the manufacturer's usage. Generally, the term *central field* refers to the central 30°, and *peripheral field* refers to the portions of visual space between 30° and 60° from fixation (and may include areas farther out, again depending on the manufacturer of the instrument). *Full field* refers to a test that includes test points centered around fixation within the central 30° and out to 60°.

Kinetic Perimetry

The term kinetic refers to motion; kinetic perimetry is a type of visual field test in which the boundaries of the visual field are determined by moving the test object while the patient's fixation is held steady. Testing is performed with test objects of fixed size and intensity (brightness), and is usually done by moving the object from areas where the patient is expected not to see them toward the center. The patient indicates that the object has entered the field of vision by some type of response: pushing a button that may cause a beep, stating "seen," or "now," etc. The perimetrist will somehow record the location where the object was first seen (discussed in Chapters 3, 4, and 5 under the various testing methods). The object is then moved to another meridian and again moved from non-seeing toward seeing. After all meridia have been tested, the perimetrist will have defined the boundary area to that particular test object. The boundary, or isopter, corresponds to a fixed height of the island of vision, and all areas within the boundary would be expected to be able to respond to the same test object plus any that are larger or brighter. Each of the lines in the bottom of Figure 1-2 represent such boundaries of equal or greater sensitivity. The classic methods of kinetic perimetry are the tangent screen and the Goldmann perimeter.

Static Perimetry

Determining the sensitivity of a visual field point by using a test object of fixed size, keeping the stimulus on the point being tested (not moving, ie, static), and increasing its intensity until it is seen is known as static perimetry. Results are usually displayed with the sensitivity plotted against the location, as shown in the top of Figure 1-2. The results for only one meridian can be displayed at a time, and correspond to a vertical cut, or profile, of the island of vision. The principle of static perimetry is used in a different format in the computerized perimeters available today. Instead of plotting sensitivity against location, today's machines are capable of graphically displaying the sensitivities on a two-dimensional grid. This gives the appearance of the island of vision in three dimensions. The application of static perimetry as used today will be discussed in detail in Chapter 5.

Manual Perimetry

Manual perimetry simply refers to the need for the perimetrist to perform all aspects of the test, including the placement and presentation of stimuli, recording of responses, and preparation of the results chart. The classic methods of manual perimetry, discussed in Chapters 3 and 4, are confrontation testing, the tangent screen, and the Goldmann perimeter. The Goldmann perimeter is capable of performing both kinetic and static perimetry, but all aspects of the test must be handled by the perimetrist.

Automated Perimetry

The more tedious aspects of perimetry may be controlled by a computer. Positioning and presentation of the stimulus, recording and keeping track of patient responses, and preparation of a printout of the results may all be computerized. The incorporation of computer technology into a visual field test is known as automated perimetry. Manufacturers of automated perimeters include Dicon, Zeiss-Humphrey, and Interzeag (makers of the Octopus™ perimeters). Automated machines are most capable of performing static perimetry, which is a very tedious process to manually perform. Automated perimetry will be discussed in Chapter 5. Static perimetry requires the patient to respond to a projected stimulus of fixed size, location, and duration at a given intensity level. In order to understand what static perimetry is measuring, it is necessary to understand the terms and units used to express the results. Some of these terms will be explained later in this chapter.

Isopter

In the discussion of kinetic perimetry, it was noted that a moving test object of fixed size and intensity defines a boundary, and sensitivity within the boundary would be expected to be equal to or greater than that

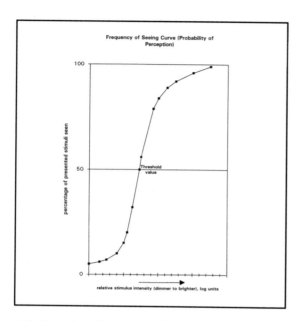

Figure 1-3. The probability of seeing a light increases as it becomes brighter.

at the boundary. Boundaries of visual field areas of equal or greater sensitivity are known as isopters ("iso" = same). The Goldmann perimeter is the classic isopter perimeter. The isopters are labeled in a way that identifies the size and intensity of the object used to define them.

Threshold

The results of a visual field test may be presented in many different formats, depending on the machine used and the available software. Common to all formats (in one form or another) is the concept of threshold. Even in kinetic perimetry, the boundary of an isopter is a threshold measurement, delineating areas capable of seeing a target (inside the line) from areas which cannot.

When a stimulus is projected against a background, the patient has only two possible responses: push the response button (implying that the stimulus was seen), or don't push the response button (implying that the stimulus was not seen). Because of the possibility of false responses, the response or lack of a response is just an implication and not actual proof that the light was seen or not seen. For a stimulus of fixed size and location, there is a certain probability (dependent on its intensity) that it will be seen. This probability can be plotted against the stimulus intensity, creating a probability of perception curve. One such hypothetical curve is shown in Figure 1-3.

For any given stimulus at a visual field point there is a certain probability that a response will be elicited, proportional to its intensity. Dim stimuli approach (but never reach) 0% probability of eliciting a response, and bright lights approach (but never reach) 100% probability. A very bright light projected into the central portion of the visual field has a very high probability of being seen, while a dim light projected into the far periphery has a very small chance of being seen. However, human beings are not perfect test subjects, and there is a certain amount of inaccuracy built into their ability to respond in a test situation. If told to push a button when presented with a light, even a blind person may on occasion think a light was seen when a dim light is presented to the periphery of the field. Similarly, a bright light projected onto the fovea of a young, healthy adult may on occasion fail to elicit a response. These considerations give rise to the definition of threshold (corresponding to the height of the island of vision at the test point). Threshold for a given point is defined as that stimulus intensity (for an object of fixed size and duration of presentation) which has a 50% probability of being seen. One important consideration based on this definition is that it is possible to obtain a different answer each time threshold is determined. In fact, this variability, known as fluctuation, is measurable in the normal population and has clinical significance.

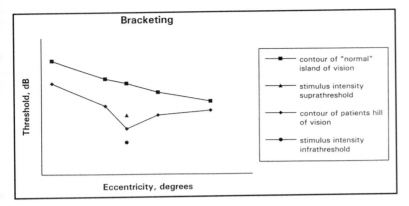

Figure 1-4. The concept of bracketing, illustrating that during the determination of threshold at a given point the stimuli will sometimes be above threshold and sometimes below. The intensity is varied according to the patient's responses.

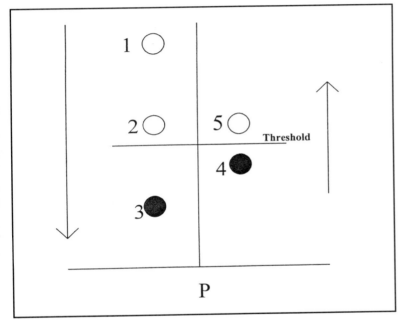

Figure 1-5. Double-crossing of threshold, the staircase method. Threshold determination at a visual field point, P. Open circles indicate patient response to stimulus; filled circles indicate no response to stimulus. Down arrow indicates stimuli decreasing in 4 dB steps; up arrow indicates stimuli increasing in 2 dB steps. Numbers indicate order of stimulus presentation.

Determination of Threshold

It would be impractical to test each point in the field with thousands of stimuli of varying intensity to find the one that is seen 50% of the time. Fortunately, an algorithm exists, which has an accuracy of +/- 1 decibel (dB, which is a measure of light intensity), 99% of the time. This algorithm varies the intensity of the presented stimuli according to the patient's response to the previous stimulus. The concepts involved are:

Bracketing

During determination of threshold at each point in the test grid, stimulus intensities will vary in such a way that some will be suprathreshold (brighter than necessary to elicit a response most of the time) and some will be infrathreshold (too dim to elicit a response most of the time). Threshold is thus "bracketed" by the test stimuli as the examination proceeds. This is illustrated in Figure 1-4.

Double Crossing of Threshold

Unless using a non-standard test strategy, stimulus intensities are varied during the test according to the patient's responses in such a manner that threshold will be crossed twice. This is illustrated in Figure 1-5. In this example, the first stimulus presented at the point P is seen (open circle, labeled "1") and the patient pushes the response button. The machine then tests that point again with a dimmer stimulus, turning down

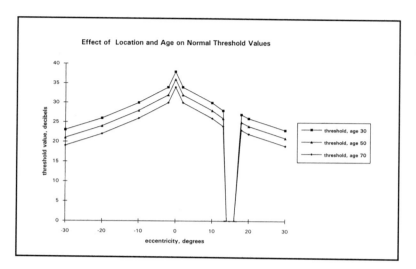

Figure 1-6. Factors influencing threshold values.

the intensity by 4 dB. This process continues (stimulus number "2" was also seen, indicated by the open circle) until the stimulus is too dim to elicit a response (stimulus "3," lack of response indicated by filled circle), ie, the intensity is now below threshold and threshold has been crossed for the first time. The machine now makes the stimulus brighter, but in two dB steps, until the patient pushes the button, indicating the second crossing of threshold (stimulus "4" was not seen; stimulus "5" was). Because the step size was 2 dB, threshold is the value that lies between the intensity values of the last two stimuli. Obviously, if the first stimulus presented at that point was not seen, the machine will make the stimulus brighter by 4 dB until threshold is first crossed and then dimmer in 2 dB steps until the second crossing. On the average, it takes five stimulus presentations at each point to determine threshold.

Random Stimulus Presentations

If the machine continually presented stimuli to one point in the field until threshold was determined, the patient would quickly learn where the next stimulus would be. Therefore, the machine tests points randomly during the course of the test. The computer keeps track of the prior responses at each point, varying the next stimulus intensity accordingly. On the Humphrey Field Analyzer™ , the point being tested will flash on the video display, and the threshold number will appear when the determination is complete.

Normal Threshold Values

Figure 1-6 illustrates the two main influences on normal threshold values—location in the field and age. Note that the most sensitive point in the field, as expected, is the fovea, corresponding to 0° of eccentricity. Sensitivity then decreases as the points move away from the center, indicated by lower threshold values. The slope of the decrease is known from studies of the normal population and is not linear, ie, the slope constantly changes from point to point. As a rough approximation, however, the sensitivity of the visual field outside of the macula (beyond 5° of eccentricity) decreases about 0.3 dB for each degree of eccentricity. This drop-off in sensitivity from the center toward the periphery is what gives the island of vision its characteristic shape. Sensitivity also decreases with age as indicated by the lower curves in the figure. The decrease is uniform across the field and is on the magnitude of 0.6 to 1 dB per point for each decade of life. As will be discussed later, because of the age-related change in threshold it is important to make sure the patient's birth date is correctly entered into the machine if the results are to be compared to an age-related normal population.

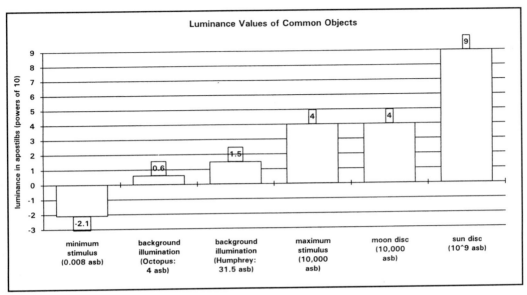

Figure 1-7. Luminance values.

Units of Measurement

Apostilb

A threshold visual field test on an automated perimeter such as the Humphrey Field Analyzer is per-formed by projecting lights into the bowl. The light reflects off the back of the bowl toward the patient's eye. The intensity of light reflecting off of a surface is expressed in units of luminance, which is a measure of light density, ie, units of light per a unit of area. Different measurement systems have led to a great deal of confusion in terminology. The apostilb (asb) is the unit used most in static threshold perimetry. One asb can be thought of as the equivalent amount of light coming off of one square centimeter of solidifying platinum at 2040° Kelvin. Figure 1-7 shows the luminance values of some common objects. Of note is the maximum stimulus intensity of the Humphrey Field Analyzer, which is roughly equivalent to the amount of light com-ing off of the full moon on a clear night. This value is 10,000 asb.

Decibel

Although measured in asb, it is not convenient to express threshold values in asb. A printout of thresh-olds expressed in asb would be difficult to read, because the sensitivity of the human visual system ranges from approximately one asb to more than 1,000,000 asb, a range of more than 6 log units (a log unit is a power of 10). A printout would therefore have numbers ranging from single digits to five digits. Fortunate-ly, the expression of luminance values on a relative scale is convenient and appropriate to the way the human visual system perceives changes in light intensity. A small change of one or a few asb, particularly in the upper end of the range (ie, brighter stimuli), is not detectable. However, the human eye is capable of detect-ing a change (brighter or dimmer) if the stimulus is changed by a power of 10 or fraction thereof. Thus, it is convenient to express threshold values in terms of a relative logarithmic scale in which the stimulus inten-sities are varied by powers of 10. The dB scale is used, in which 1 dB is equal to one tenth of a log unit. The dB scale expresses threshold as a fraction of the maximum available stimulus intensity; that is, it measures how much the maximum available stimulus intensity was attenuated (dimmed) until threshold was deter-mined using the above algorithm. It is important to realize that the asb value expressed by the dB number is relative to the maximum available stimulus intensity on a particular instrument and will thus vary from one

Table 1-1
Decibel/Apostilb/Goldmann Equivalents

Intensity		Actual Humphrey Test Stimulus Size				
dB	Asb	I	II	III	IV	V
0	10,000	III4e	IV4e	V4e		
1	7,943	III4d	IV4d	V4d		
2	6,310	III4c	III4c	V4c		
3	5,012	III4b	IV4b	V4b		
4	3,981	III4a	IV4a	V4a		
5	3,162	II4e	III4e	IV4e	V4e	
6	2,512	II4d	III4d	IV4d	V4d	
7	1,995	II4c	III4c	III4c	V4c	
8	1,585	II4b	III4b	IV4b	V4b	
9	1,259	II4a	III4a	IV4a	V4a	
10	1,000	I4e	II4e	III4e	IV4e	V4e
11	794	I4d	II4d	III4d	IV4d	V4d
12	631	I4c	II4c	III4c	III4c	V4c
13	501	I4b	II4b	III4b	IV4b	V4b
14	398	I4a	II4a	III4a	IV4a	V4a
15	316	I3e	II3e	III3e	IV3e	V3e
16	251	I3d	II3d	III3d	IV3d	V3d
17	200	I3c	II3c	III3c	IV3c	V3c
18	158	I3d	II3b	III3b	IV3b	V3b
19	126	I3a	II3a	III3a	IV3a	V3a
20	100	I2e	II2e	III2e	IV2e	V2e
21	79	I2d	II2d	III2d	IV2d	V2d
22	63	I2c	II2c	III2c	IV2c	V2c
23	50	I2b	II2b	III2b	IV2b	V2b
24	40	I2a	II2a	III2a	IV2a	V2a
25	32	I1e	III1e	III1e	IV1e	V1e
26	25	I1d	III1d	III1d	IV1d	V1d
27	20	I1c	III1c	III1c	IV1c	V1c
28	16	I1b	III1b	III1b	IV1b	V1b
29	13	I1a	III1a	III1a	IV1a	V1a
30	10		I1e	I2e	III1e	IV1e
31	8		I1d	I2d	III1d	IV1d
32	6		I1c	I2c	III1c	IV1c
33	5		I1b	I2b	III1b	IV1b
34	4		I1a	I2a	III1a	IV1a
35	3.2			I1e	I2e	III1e
36	2.5			I1d	I2d	III1d
37	2.0			I1c	I2c	III1c
38	1.6			I1b	I2b	III1b
39	1.3			I1a	I2a	III1a
40	1.0				I1e	I2e
41	0.8				I1d	I2d
42	0.6				I1c	I2c
43	0.5				I1b	I2b

Intensity		Actual Humphrey Test Stimulus Size				
dB	Asb	I	II	III	IV	V
44	0.4				I1a	I2a
45	0.32					I1e
46	0.25					I1d
47	0.20					I1c
48	0.16					I1b
49	0.13					I1a
50	0.10					I4e
51	0.08					I4d

Table 1-1 (continued)
Decibel/Apostilb/Goldmann Equivalents

perimeter to another if the maximum available stimulus intensities are different. The Humphrey Field Analyzer changes the stimulus intensity by interposing filters of increasing density in front of the projector bulb.

To illustrate the relationship between light intensity expressed in asb and dB, assume the maximum available stimulus intensity is 10,000, or 10^4 asb, as is the case with the Humphrey Field Analyzer. If the brightest available stimulus was determined to be the threshold value at a point, it would be represented by 0 dB. A "0" would appear on the printout of threshold values. Threshold values less than zero (ie, the patient failed to respond to the maximum stimulus intensity) would be indicated by "<0." If the threshold value was recorded as "1," this would mean that the 10,000 asb maximum available stimulus was dimmed by 0.1 log units. The asb value of this stimulus would be $10^{4-0.1}$, or $10^{3.9}$, which equals 7,943 asb. Similarly, dimming of the maximum available stimulus by 4 dB (indicated by a "4" on the value table printout) would mean that threshold was equal to $10^{4-(0.1\times4)}$, or $10^{3.6}$, which equals 3,981 asb. Note that the dB scale is linear (ie, changes in units), while the asb scale is not. Table 1-1 relates dB, asb, and Goldmann equivalents.

It is important to realize that as the dB numbers increase on a value table printout, the maximum available stimulus intensity is being turned down by an increasing amount. Threshold corresponding to a dimmer stimulus means greater retinal sensitivity. Thus, on a value table printout (the report of the patient's actual measured thresholds) larger dB values correspond to better sensitivity, and smaller dB numbers indicate loss of sensitivity.

The Goldmann stimulus labels will be discussed in Chapter 4. The conversion information shown in Table 1-1 is useful if a visual field test with a specific Goldmann target is required, as is sometimes specified by state disability examinations, for example. Most automated perimeters may be set to test with a stimulus of fixed intensity, which may be selected based on the equivalent Goldmann stimulus shown in the table.

Types of Visual Field Defects

Scotoma

Visual field loss means an alteration in the height and shape of the island of vision. Points in the field will show decreases in sensitivity from the levels they should have (alteration of height) and will not show the expected changes from neighboring points due to eccentricity (alteration of shape). Figure 1-8 illustrates common visual field defects as recorded by static threshold techniques on an automated perimeter. The top curve of the figure represents a profile of a "normal" island of vision for a person of a certain age. The middle curve is from a patient with a disease process that diffusely affects all points in the visual field. Note that

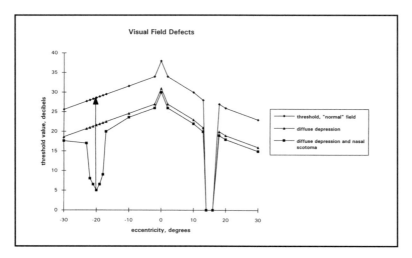

Figure 1-8. Types of visual field defects as recorded by automated static perimetry.

the shape of the curve is the same as the normal island but that all of the points manifest a uniform decrease in sensitivity. This is called diffuse depression, or "generalized reduction in sensitivity." If this field was mapped with isopter perimetry on a Goldmann perimeter, all of the isopters would appear smaller than they should, with the circumferences of the isopters moved toward the center of the plot. This is known as "constriction" of the visual field and is thus analogous to diffuse depression as recorded on static threshold perimetry. Factors that influence the visual field to produce such diffuse loss of sensitivity will be discussed in subsequent chapters.

The lower curve in Figure 1-8 shows diffuse depression as well but also shows additional loss centered around 20° nasally. This additional depression is known as focal loss, or a scotoma. Webster's defines a scotoma as "an area of pathologically diminished vision within the visual field."

Because threshold information is quantitative, it is possible to determine the exact amount of sensitivity loss at each point by subtracting the patient's measured threshold value from that of the expected normal value. This is known as the defect depth and is expressed in dB. The larger the defect depth, the more pathological the field. The arrow in Figure 1-8 indicates the defect depth for the scotoma at 20° nasally. Because the visual field exhibits a combination of diffuse loss and focal loss, if one wanted to determine the extent of the focal loss only, it would be necessary to "correct" the island of vision for the diffuse loss by raising all of the threshold values by an amount equal to the average diffuse loss. Following such correction, any defects left over would represent focal loss.

Defects can be characterized by the magnitude of their depth—those between 5 dB and 9 dB from expected are "shallow," 10 dB to 19 dB may be considered moderate, defects over 20 dB are deep, and thresholds less than the maximum available stimulus intensity are considered "absolute." It should be pointed out that the measurement of an absolute defect does not necessarily mean total loss of sensitivity—it only means that the machine was not capable of generating a stimulus bright enough to elicit a response.

Examples of focal visual field defects that could be seen in the central 30° of a right eye are illustrated in Figure 1-9. These include the central scotoma (Figure 1-9a), the centrocecal scotoma, which involves the central vision and the blind spot (Figure 1-9b), the nasal step (Figure 1-9c), paracentral scotoma (Figure 1-9d), arcuate scotoma (Figure 1-9e), and the nerve fiber bundle defect (Figure 1-9f). The physiologic blind spot is the vertical oval located to the right of the vertical meridian in 1-9a, c, and d. Because it connects to the scotoma it is said to be involved in situations 1-9b, e, and f.

Hemianopia

Hemianopia is a special visual field term that refers to loss of one half of the visual field in one or both eyes ("hemi" = half). Hemianopic defects are illustrated in Figure 1-10.

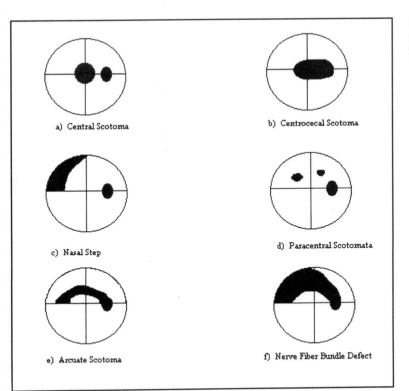

Figure 1-9. Types of monocular visual field defects.

a) Central Scotoma

b) Centrocecal Scotoma

c) Nasal Step

d) Paracentral Scotomata

e) Arcuate Scotoma

f) Nerve Fiber Bundle Defect

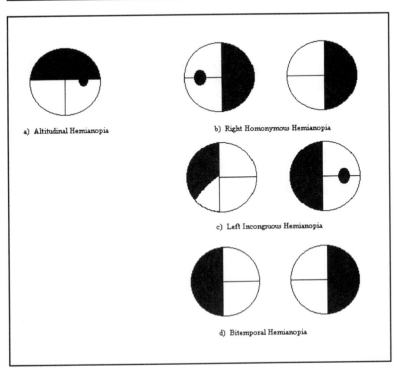

Figure 1-10. Hemianopic visual field defects.

a) Altitudinal Hemianopia

b) Right Homonymous Hemianopia

c) Left Incongruous Hemianopia

d) Bitemporal Hemianopia

If the upper or lower half of the field is lost, respecting the horizontal midline, the loss is termed an altitudinal hemianopia (Figure 1-10a). Hemianopic loss respecting the vertical midline usually does not occur in one eye only, because this type of loss is due to disease at the chiasm or even more posteriorly where fibers from both eyes will be involved. (This is explained in Chapter 2.) Thus the terms nasal or temporal hemianopia are not used. Loss occurring on the same side of the vertical midline in each eye is called a homonymous hemianopia and is designated by the involved side. Figure 1-10b illustrates a right homonymous hemianopia. If the loss is fairly symmetrical between the two eyes it is said to be congruous; the more posterior the lesion causing the loss, the more congruous the loss. Figure 1-10c illustrates a left incongruous hemianopia due to a lesion located just behind the optic chiasm. Finally, a hemianopia that involves the temporal field in each eye is called a bitemporal hemianopia, illustrated in Figure 1-10d. Binasal hemianopias are very unusual and rarely encountered.

Chapter 2

Anatomic Basis for the Visual Field

KEY POINTS

- The anatomy of the visual system forms the basis for visual field defects.

- Because axons do not cross the horizontal raphe, lesions of the optic disc produce visual field defects that do not cross the horizontal meridian.

- Lesions in the visual pathway anterior to the optic chiasm produce monocular visual field defects; lesions of the chiasm or posterior to it produce visual field defects manifesting in both eyes.

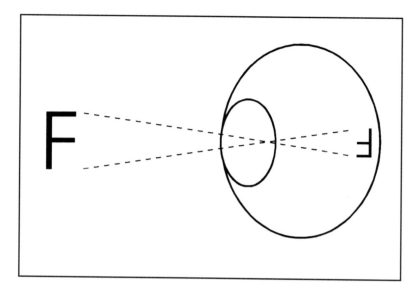

Figure 2-1. Images on the retina are inverted and reversed.

OptA
OptT
OphA
OphT
CL
Optn

Introduction

The visual pathway consists of nerve fibers, or axons, which connect the retina to the visual cortex of the occipital lobes in the brain. In their route to the visual cortex, the nerve fibers pass from the retina to the optic disc. After passing through the optic disc, they join together to become the optic nerve as it traverses the orbit into the cranium to enter the optic chiasm. From there, visual information passes to the lateral geniculate ganglion and then to the occipital cortex.

An understanding of the anatomy of the visual system guides the clinician to proper visual field test selection as well as in the interpretation of the findings. At times, the patterns of visual field loss can precisely localize the causative lesion. These patterns are the result of the path that visual neurons take as they traverse from the retina to the occipital cortex. A review of the visual pathways will help the reader understand the importance of the visual field in locating lesions of the afferent visual system.

Images must reach the retina before they can be converted into neurological signals for transmission to the brain. The eye's optical system consists primarily of the precorneal tear film, the cornea, and the crystalline lens, as well as any corrective spectacle or contact lenses which may be in place. By virtue of the optics of this system, images created by it are inverted on the retina, that is, upside down and reversed left to right (Figure 2-1). Objects that lie above in visual space are imaged on the lower retina; objects below are imaged on the upper retina. Similarly, objects lying to the left in visual space have their images created on the right hand side of the retina, and objects that lie to the right create images to the left of the center of the retina.

OptA
OptT
OphA
OphT

Retina

The retina is composed of three layers of nerve cells. Images focused on the retina stimulate the outer layer consisting of the light sensitive rods and cones. The rods and cones capture the image and convert it into an electrochemical signal. This signal is passed to the middle layer of bipolar, amacrine, and horizontal cells where some processing of the information occurs. The axons, or nerve fibers, of the bipolar and amacrine cells connect to the ganglion cells in the inner layer of neural cells.

Axons of the ganglion cells form the nerve fiber layer and travel to the optic disc where they come together to form the optic nerve. Figure 2-2 illustrates the layout of these various neurons in the retina.

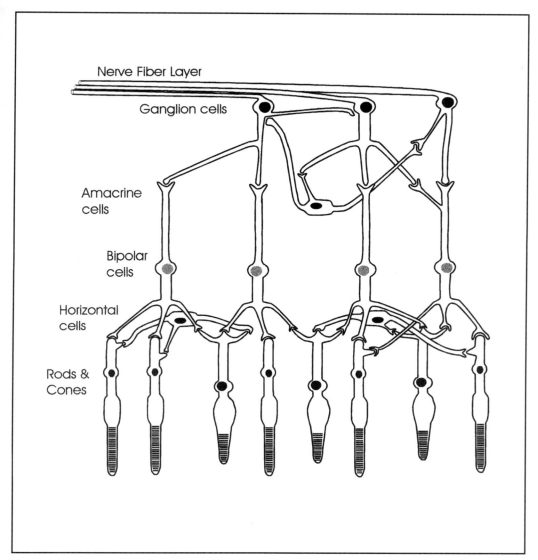

Figure 2-2. Arrangement of neurons in the retina.

The fovea is a specialized area in the retina that serves to provide sharp central vision. This region has no blood vessels within it and consists primarily of cones and their neural connections. The center of the fovea is the point of fixation for the eye and serves as a reference for the nasal, temporal, superior, and inferior visual field. Lesions in the fovea usually result in decreased visual acuity and central scotomas.

Nerve Fiber Layer and Optic Disc

The axons of the ganglion cells in the retina course toward the optic disc in the nerve fiber layer as illustrated in Figure 2-3. Fibers originating in the inferior retina (serving the superior visual field) enter the disc inferiorly, while fibers originating in the superior retina (serving the inferior visual field) enter the disc supe-

OptA
OptT
OphA
OphT

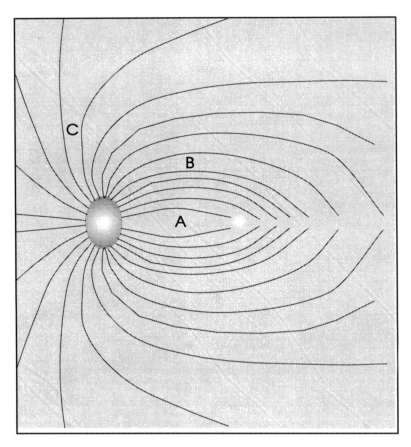

Figure 2-3. (A) The axons that travel in a direct path from the macula to the temporal side of the optic disc comprise the papillomacular bundle. Damage to these neurons results in central or cecocentral scotomas. (B) Axons that originate from ganglion cells temporal to the macula must travel superior or inferior to the macula in a curving fashion and enter the optic disc at the superior and inferior poles; these axons make up the arcuate fibers. Damage to axons in the arcuate bundle leads to nasal step field defects, Bjerrum, paracentral, and arcuate scotomas. (C) Axons that originate in the nasal retina travel in a mostly radial fashion and enter the disc nasally. Damage to these fibers gives rise to wedge defects. The nerve fibers do not cross the horizontal raphe.

riorly. Neurons originating temporal to the fovea (serving the nasal visual field) enter the optic disc at the superior and inferior poles, bending around the macula in arcuate bundles. Axons originating nasal to the fovea (serving the temporal visual field) enter the disc on the nasal and temporal sides, with the papillomacular bundle entering the disc on its temporal side. No fibers cross over the horizontal raphe, a demarcation separating the inferior and superior halves of the retina.

The optic disc lies about 3 mm nasal to the fovea and is 1 mm wide and 1½ mm high. There are no photoreceptors overlying the optic disc, so images projected onto the optic disc are not seen. This is the physiologic blind spot, and is approximately 5.5° wide and 7.5° high and lies 15° temporal to fixation in the field. Figure 2-4 illustrates the location of the physiologic blind spot and how its size varies with distance from the eye. Because axons do not cross the horizontal raphe, lesions of the optic disc produce visual field defects that do not cross the horizontal meridian.

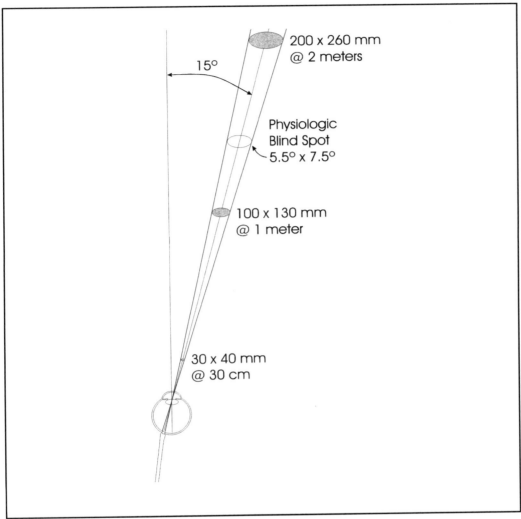

Figure 2-4. Projection of the physiologic blind spot into visual space.

Optic Nerve

The neurons enter the optic disc in bundles to pass through the pores in the lamina cribrosa, the specialized area of the sclera where the optic nerve exits the eye. As they traverse the optic nerve on their path toward the optic chiasm, the macular fibers move to a more central location in the nerve. The axons tend to maintain the temporal-nasal and superior-inferior relationship that began in the retina. Because large numbers of neurons carry macular information, lesions of the optic nerve tend to produce unilateral central field defects, but other patterns are often seen.

Optic Chiasm

The optic chiasm is that portion of the visual pathway where the optic nerves from the two eyes come together. Here the fibers mix together in a special pattern. Axons that originate nasal to the fovea cross to

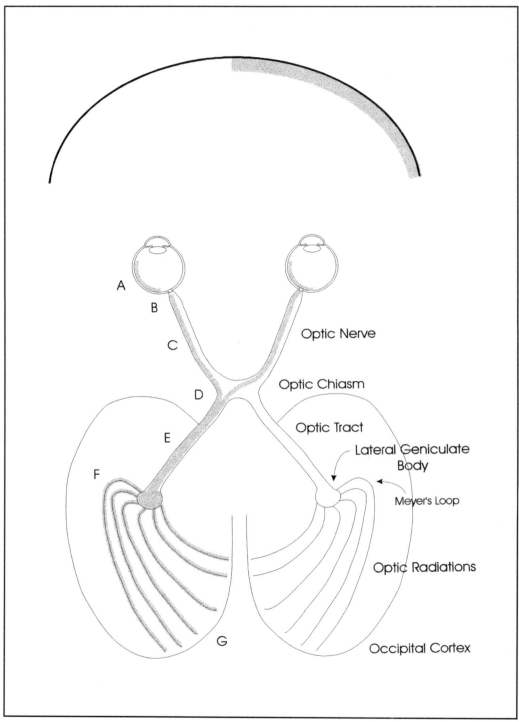

Figure 2-5. The visual pathway. The path of an image on the right side is depicted in gray. At the optic chiasm, neurons from the right eye (carrying information from the right field) cross to the left side and join with the neurons from the left eye (also carrying information from the right field). The letters on the left side of the figure coorespond to lesions that produce the visual fields in Figures 2-6 to 2-12.

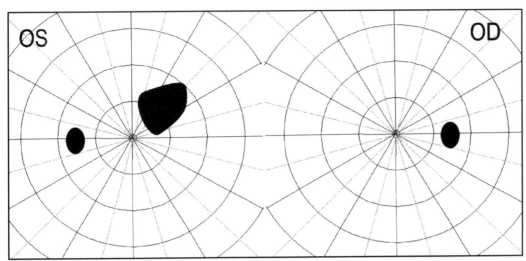

Figure 2-6. Visual field defect arising from a retinal lesion (point A in Figure 2-5).

the opposite side, while those from the temporal side continue their path without crossing. This partial crossing of fibers is called a hemidecussation and is illustrated in Figure 2-5. Thus the visual pathway behind the chiasm consists of fibers carrying images from the nasal field from the same side and the temporal field from the opposite side. This arrangement allows the right side of the brain to perceive images from the left visual field and the left side of the brain to perceive images from the right side. The crossing fibers in the chiasm are more sensitive to injury; lesions in the chiasm usually affect the temporal visual field in each eye.

Intracranial Pathway

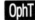

After leaving the optic chiasm, the axons continue posteriorly as the optic tracts until reaching the lateral geniculate body. There they synapse with the cells whose axons are destined for the occipital cortex. The axons leaving the lateral geniculate fan out in the optic radiations. Some of the inferior fibers bend around the temporal horn of the lateral ventricle into the temporal lobe on their way to the inferior portion of the occipital pole. These fibers are known as Meyer's loop. The superior fibers take a more direct route through the parietal lobe, finally reaching the superior portion of the occipital pole. Macular fibers project onto the tip and over the outer surface of the occipital cortex, while the fibers serving the peripheral visual field terminate on either side of the calcarine fissure on the medial surface of the occipital lobes.

Posterior to the optic chiasm, the fibers from one side no longer represent the eye on that side, but rather the visual space from the opposite side. Lesions in the visual pathways behind the chiasm produce field defects on one side of both eyes. These defects, known as homonymous hemianopias, do not cross the vertical meridian. As they course posteriorly, fibers representing adjacent visual space get closer together; therefore visual field defects in each eye tend to become more alike (congruous) the closer the lesion is to the occipital lobe. Even with total loss of the fibers on one side, good acuity is maintained because half of the macular fibers are uninvolved (ie, those from the other side).

Correlation of Anatomy and Visual Field Loss

Examination of the visual field is performed to detect damage, survey its extent, determine the location of the damage, and guide therapy. Damage to or abnormalities in the visual pathways can arise from a vari-

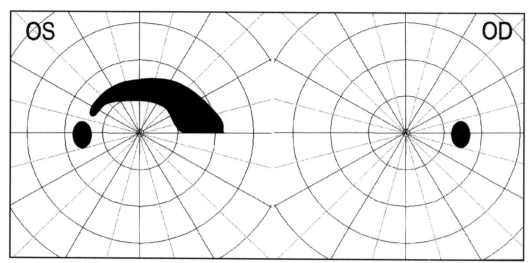

Figure 2-7. Arcuate scotoma arising from an optic disc based lesion, such as would be seen in glaucoma (point B in Figure 2-5).

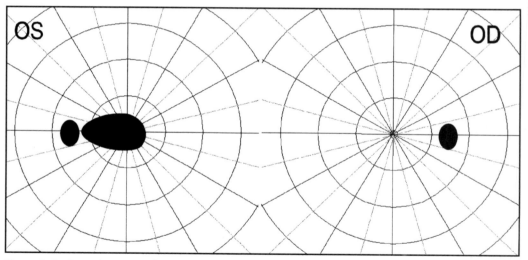

Figure 2-8. Central scotoma from an optic nerve lesion (point C in Figure 2-5). If the physiologic blind spot was included in the scotoma, it would be termed cecocentral.

ety of causes. Congenital defects, genetic disorders, inflammations, infections, tumors, trauma, and metabolic and circulatory abnormalities can all lead to detectable visual field abnormalities. With an understanding of ocular anatomy, the perimetrist and clinician can know where to look for lesions that have resulted in visual field defects.

Artifactual field loss from external obstructions, discussed in detail in Chapter 3, does not respect the horizontal or vertical meridians. These boundaries are determined by the horizontal raphe in the nerve fiber layer and the hemidecussation in the optic chiasm. Retinal lesions are usually visible with the ophthalmoscope and produce field defects that correspond in size and shape to the lesion (Figure 2-6). Optic disc-based lesions usually result in nasal steps, Bjerrum scotomas, arcuate defects, altitudinal losses, or temporal wedge defects. Figure 2-7 demonstrates a typical disc-based arcuate scotoma.

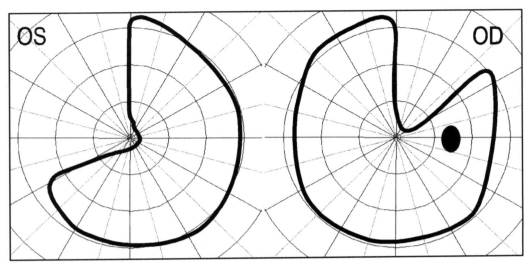

Figure 2-9. Bitemporal defect typical for chiasmal lesions (point D in Figure 2-5). Note that the defect commonly includes a central scotoma in the more involved eye, as is seen in the left eye in this example.

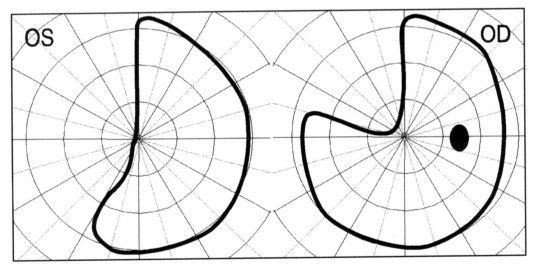

Figure 2-10. Incongruous incomplete left hemianopia arising from a lesion at point E in Figure 2-5 in the right optic tract.

Optic nerve lesions classically produce cecocentral or central scotomas, as shown in Figure 2-8. At the optic chiasm, visual space is divided anatomically into right and left halves. Lesions involving the chiasm usually result in visual field defects involving the temporal field in both eyes (Figure 2-9). Lesions in the pathways posterior to the chiasm result in field defects in each eye on the side opposite the lesion. Visual field defects arising from lesions at or behind the chiasm do not cross the vertical meridian of the field (unless multiple lesions are present and both sides are involved). The nearer a posterior pathway lesion is to the occipital cortex, the more congruous, or similar, are the defects in each eye. Figure 2-10 depicts a typical field for a lesion in the left optic tract. Notice that the visual field defect is incongruous, or more extensive in one eye than the other. Lesions in the posterior temporal lobes produce superior visual field defects

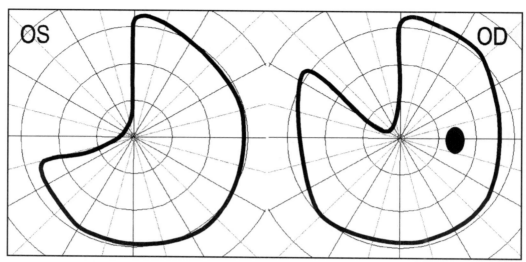

Figure 2-11. This slightly more congruous incomplete superior hemianopia results from a lesion in Meyer's loop (point F in Figure 2-5).

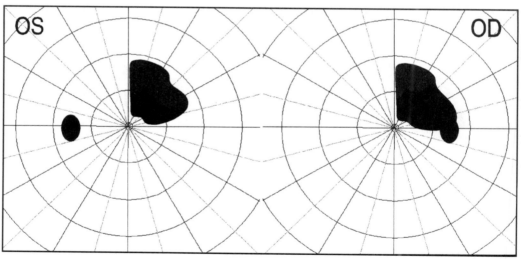

Figure 2-12. Highly congruous homonymous field defect resulting from an occipital cortex lesion (point G in Figure 2-5).

like the one in Figure 2-11 because of damage to the neurons in Meyer's loop. Injury to the occipital cortex results in highly congruous visual field defects like the one shown in Figure 2-12.

Section II

METHODS OF TESTING THE VISUAL FIELD

Chapter 3

Basic Methods

- Simple methods of visual field testing exist that are not dependent on costly or complex machines.

- Confrontation testing may rapidly uncover visual field defects.

- The Amsler grid can be used to explore patient complaints related to the central vision and macular disease.

- The tangent screen provides a relatively inexpensive method for testing the central 30°.

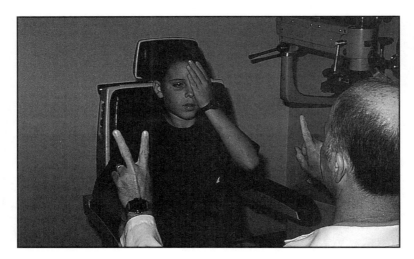

Figure 3-1. Correct position of examiner and patient for confrontation testing. The examiner closes his or her eye directly opposite the patient's occluded eye.

Introduction

There are many methods and devices available for measuring the visual field. The methods described in this chapter are not dependent on costly or complex machines. They employ simple, inexpensive, and usually rapid means for detecting and quantifying visual field defects.

Confrontation Visual Field Testing

The most basic type of visual field testing is confrontation. Because it is simple and requires no equipment, it can be performed nearly anywhere, anytime—in the clinic, at the bedside, or in the emergency department. Confrontation visual field testing is a rapid screening method for visual field defects. In addition to simple detection of visual field defects, confrontation testing can also be used to estimate the extent of visual field defects. Even under the most controlled circumstances, this method is only semi-quantitative and detects only gross field defects, so patients who demonstrate abnormalities on confrontation testing should undergo quantitative perimetry. Circumstances where confrontation testing is useful include screening during a routine eye exam, examination of non-verbal patients, and examination of patients suspected of malingering.

Technique

The examiner and patient face each other, about 1 m apart. No spectacle correction is necessary if the patient's uncorrected vision is at least finger counting at 3 ft. If it is not, have the patient wear his or her usual spectacles. The patient is instructed to cover the left eye with his or her own hand. The examiner closes his or her own right eye, so that the open eyes of the examiner and patient are opposite each other. This allows the examiner to use his or her own field as a check against the patient's. The patient is instructed to look at the examiner's nose. The examiner's fingers are presented in a plane halfway between the examiner and the patient in all four quadrants. The patient is asked to indicate when and how many fingers are seen. Figure 3-1 depicts the technique.

By comparing the patient's answers with what the examiner sees, normalcy can be determined and gross visual field defects detected. To speed up this already quick process, fingers can be simultaneously presented in both inferior or superior quadrants and the patient can be asked to report the total number seen. If a patent has difficulty with simultaneous presentations but the field appears normal to single presentations, there may be a lesion in the parietal lobe. It is best to use one, two, or five fingers as test targets, because it is more difficult to quickly count three or four fingers in the peripheral field. After the right eye is tested, the patient's left eye is examined in a similar manner, switching the occluded eyes of both examiner and patient.

What the Patient Needs to Know

- This is a test of your side vision, or what you see around and to the sides.

- Each eye is checked separately. Please keep the other eye covered.

- Look at my nose at all times. I'll be asking you questions about my hands, but they will be in your side vision. Don't look at my hand. Keep looking at my nose.

When a field defect is detected using finger counting confrontation, some measurement of its extent can be made by presenting a small target, such as a cotton tipped applicator, in the area of abnormality and noting where the patient first sees it. The defect can be mapped and the size estimated in degrees of field loss.

The results of confrontation testing are documented as follows: if the field appears normal, record that the field is full to confrontation. For example, "VF - FTC OU" means "visual field full to confrontation in both eyes." If there is an abnormality, record it in words (for example, "VF - difficulty CF infero-temporal quadrant OS") or draw a simple diagram depicting the abnormality.

Elicited eye movements can be used to test the visual field in non-verbal patients. An unexpected object, a threatening gesture, a light, or a toy can be presented in each quadrant. Eye movements toward or aversion from the stimulus suggest a grossly intact visual field in the quadrant tested.

Amsler Grid Testing

The Amsler grid is a tool for evaluating the macular region of the central visual field. It is used when there is decreased vision and when the patient reports distortion of vision or a small scotoma in the central vision. Macular diseases, such as age-related macular degeneration and central serous retinopathy, as well as some optic nerve disorders, commonly give rise to abnormalities that can be detected using the Amsler grid.

The standard chart consists of a grid printed on a flat black card. The lines are 5 mm apart and the entire grid measures 10 cm. The center of the grid has a white spot for fixation. Figure 3-2 is an example of the standard Amsler grid chart.

When used at a testing distance of 28 cm to 30 cm, the grid represents approximately the central 10° of the visual field. Figure 3-3 depicts the grid projected onto the retina. As can be seen, the Amsler grid covers the macular region of the retina. The temporal edge of the chart lies about 5° from the physiologic blind spot.

Additional charts are available for special circumstances. For patients who have lost central vision, a chart is available with white diagonal lines overlying the standard grid pattern. The patient is asked to fixate at the point where the diagonal lines would appear to cross. This chart is shown in Figure 3-4.

A chart with a grid composed of red lines on the black background is available to locate shallow central and paracentral scotomas. Other charts come in the standard package; the reader is urged to consult the instructions that accompany the chart manual to learn when and how to use the less commonly used charts.

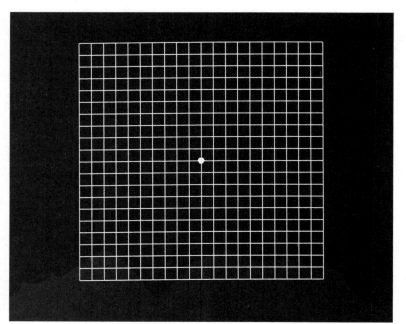

Figure 3-2. The standard Amsler grid chart.

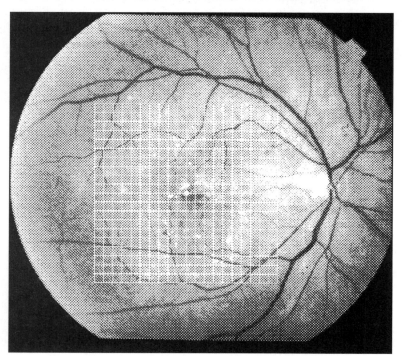

Figure 3-3. Projection of the Amsler grid over the retina.

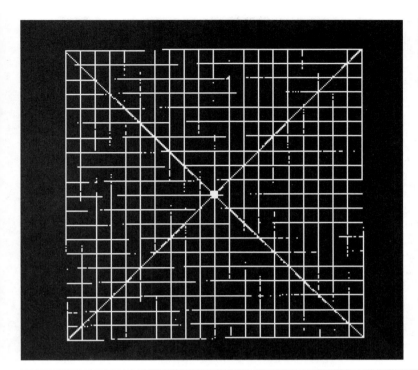

Figure 3-4. Amsler grid with diagonals for testing patients with central scotomas.

What the Patient Needs to Know

- This test is to check your side vision that is just next to your central vision and part of your central vision.

- If you use reading glasses or bifocals, please put them on.

- Hold the chart at your normal reading distance, just as you would a magazine.

- We check one eye at a time. Please keep the cover in place until I tell you.

- Look at the central dot at all times. I'll be asking questions about the rest of the grid, but you are to look only at the dot in the middle. If you cannot see the dot, do your best to look at the center of the grid.

Testing Technique

The patient should be seated comfortably. The test should be performed prior to dilation. The chart is held 28 cm to 30 cm from the patient. If the patient is aphakic, pseudophakic, or presbyopic, use the proper add for the testing distance (+3.50 diopters). If using the patient's bifocals, the test distance may be modified for the bifocal working distance. Avoid ophthalmoscopy or shining other bright lights into the patient's eyes immediately prior to administering the test, as the bright light can leave the patient with a transient central scotoma that can interfere with the test. The room illumination should be adequate for reading. Have the patient look toward the center of the card. The patient is then asked the following questions:

1. *Can you see the white spot in the center of the grid?* If the spot is not visible, the patient has a central scotoma. Show the patient the chart with diagonal lines and have the patient look at their point of intersection in the center. Instruct the patient to look at the center of the chart during the remainder of the test.

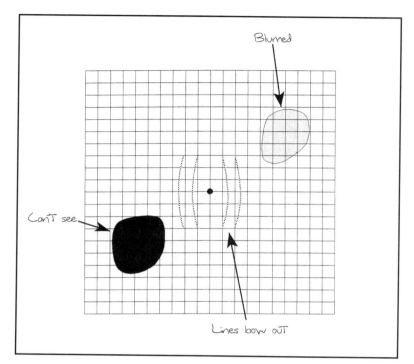

Figure 3-5. Possible results of Amsler grid testing.

2. *Keeping your gaze fixed in the center of the grid, can you see the entire grid? All four corners and all four sides?* If the answer is no, there is an edge scotoma. Have the patient point to the missing region(s).

3. *While keeping your gaze fixed in the center of the grid, is the entire grid intact? Are there any areas missing? Is it blurred anywhere?* Have the patient point out the missing or blurred areas.

4. *While keeping your gaze fixed in the center of the grid, do all the lines, both horizontal and vertical, appear straight and parallel? Are there any areas where the lines bow in or out?* Again have the patient point out the abnormal areas.

5. *3* Again have the patient point out the abnormal areas. (The term for such phenomenon is metamorphopsia.)

6. Repeat questions 2 and 3 using the red-on-black grid if shallow central or paracentral scotomas are suspected, for example in a patient with mildly blurred central vision, or as a part of an exam for drug-induced maculopathy or optic neuropathy.

Recording the Results

The results of Amsler grid testing are usually recorded on a black grid with a white background, although the examiner can draw the abnormalities (described by the patient) freehand as well. The examiner or the patient can outline scotomata and indicate where distortions or other abnormalities occur. It is useful to have the patient note the number of normal boxes between the fixation point and the region of abnormality, as well as use the boxes to indicate the extent of the abnormality. Figure 3-5 illustrates a variety of abnormalities that can be found on Amsler grid testing.

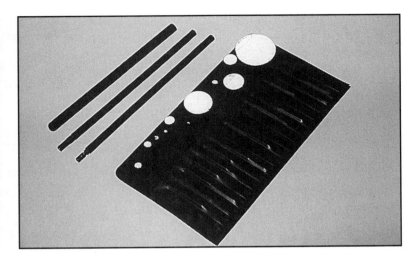

Figure 3-6. Tangent screen test objects and segmented test wand.

The Tangent Screen

The tangent screen is a good method for exploring the central 30° of the visual field. Although the equipment used is simple and inexpensive, it remains the one of the most flexible methods of visual field testing. While it is not valid to compare tangent screen results obtained at different facilities for subtle changes because of variations in testing circumstances and technique, results from serial testing in a given facility can accurately chart a patient's progress. Because the examiner is positioned between the patient and the testing surface, patient reliability is easily determined. Due to variations in testing circumstances and techniques, the tangent screen is not as useful for following the progress of chronic eye diseases as other methods such as Goldmann or automated perimetry.

The tangent screen is a flat board, usually covered with black felt. Most commercially available tangent screens measure 1 m by 1 m, and are designed for testing at a distance of 1 m. A 2 m by 2 m screen allows more flexibility for distant testing, and provides for less visual distraction when used at closer distances. The screen may be cleaned by gentle whisking.

A white button or similar target in the center of the screen serves as a fixation target. (Two pieces of white tape can be used to form a large "X" on the screen for patients with a central scotoma. The X crosses at the fixation point, and the patient is instructed to look where the lines meet in the center.) Most screens have black stitching in 5°, 10°, 15°, 20°, and 25° circles from the center, as well as radial meridians every 15°. There is also stitching to indicate where the normal blind spot should be. The patient is instructed to look at the fixation mark as a target is moved along the meridian.

As much as possible, the testing area should be free of "visual clutter" and other distractions. Illumination of the tangent screen should be even, with lighting from both sides, and ideally should provide about 7-ft candles of light on the screen. This can be measured with a standard light meter. A well-lit room with two or more light sources (to provide even illumination across the screen without shadows) is generally adequate. It is helpful if the intensity of the room illumination can be adjusted to permit variation in stimulus intensity, as subtle scotomas may be more readily detected with dimmer stimuli.

A variety of methods may be employed to check the testing distance (usually 1 meter). A black ribbon or string attached to the central fixation button permits accurate verification of the distance, as well as providing a good visual check on the patient's height relative to the fixation target. Knots or other markings can be used to indicate the standard testing distances along the ribbon. Marks on the floor or a tape measure are other alternatives.

A wide variety of targets can be used in tangent screen perimetry. Round painted discs of varying sizes, white or red on one side and flat black on the other, are the standard targets (Figure 3-6). Other colors are optional. The test target set should contain some pairs of targets where one target is twice the size of the other in the pair. These discs are attached to a wand (one at a time) and presented against the surface of the tangent screen. Disks must be replaced if they become discolored.

Disks constructed from heavy paper are easily replaced when worn or faded. Beads of various sizes can also be used. Bead targets can be attached to cloth-covered wands just below the end of the wand; rotation of the wand allows for static presentations. The Lumiwand® is a commercially available stimulus consisting of a light source that produces a uniform illumination over its surface. The intensity and color of this stimulus are voltage dependent, and the stimulus size is varied by means of caps that are placed over the lit end of the wand.

Testing Technique

Setting up

Position the patient 1 m (or other selected distance) from the tangent screen. Be sure the patient is seated comfortably. The eyes should be level with the fixation button. Use the patient's distance refraction for the correcting lens. If the patient is dilated, aphakic, pseudophakic, or presbyopic, use the proper add for the testing distance (+1.00 diopter for 1 m, +0.50 diopter for 2 m). If testing through the patient's spectacles, be sure the bifocal does not interfere with testing the inferior field. This can be easily missed if the patient wears progressive bifocals. To avoid the bifocal portion, tip the patient's chin down while testing the inferior field; this ensures that the upper part of the glasses is being used. Occlude the eye not being tested.

What the Patient Needs to Know

- This is a test of your peripheral or side vision.

- We will check one eye at a time, so one eye will be covered.

- Your job is to look at this central button during the entire test. You can blink whenever you want. As you look at the button, I'll be bringing this little dot from where you can't see it, toward you to where you can see it. When you first notice the dot, say the word "see." The trick is not to look for the dot. Keep your eye on the button all the time.

- Sometimes you'll see the dot right away. Just let me know that you see it.

- If the dot disappears, say "gone."

- The main thing is to keep your eye on the center button.

Explain the test to the patient and agree on a system of signals to indicate when the target is seen and when it disappears. It is our practice to have the patient say "see" when the target is seen and "gone" when it disappears. Make sure the patient understands that the target will appear in various places in the peripheral field and may disappear as well. Position yourself so that you can observe the patient and monitor fixation. Figure 3-7 shows a patient and examiner ready to begin testing.

Testing the Patient

For routine testing, first locate the physiologic blind spot and demonstrate it to the patient. This reinforces the explanation of the test and permits the patient some practice. Use a moderately large white target, 10 mm to 20 mm in diameter. This target should be seen easily in the periphery and will disappear when moved into the blind spot. Remind the patient to indicate when the target disappears and when it reappears.

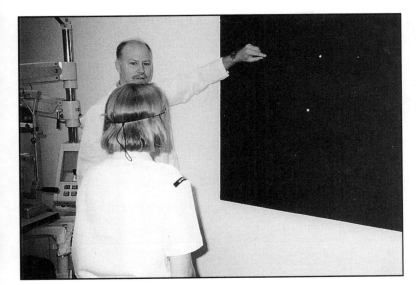

Figure 3-7. Correct position of examiner and patient for tangent screen testing. The examiner faces the patient and constantly monitors fixation.

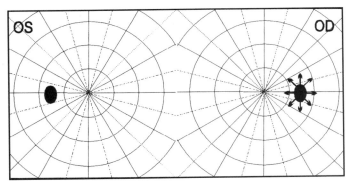

Figure 3-8. Mapping the blind spot. The target is moved from within the physiologic blind spot until seen. This is repeated in eight cardinal directions.

After demonstrating the blind spot to the patient, proceed to map it. Select a smaller target. The exact size will depend on such factors as patient acuity and alertness. It should be just large enough to be seen at 20° to 25° temporal to fixation; usually a 2 to 5 mm white test object will suffice. Place the target in the blind spot and move it out slowly in each of eight equally spaced directions, noting when the target is first seen. This location is marked by placing a black-tipped pin at the "seen" point. Figure 3-8 illustrates mapping the blind spot.

Temporary recording of the patient's responses is made on the screen itself. Black push-pins make convenient markers, as do small pieces of black felt made with a hole punch. Black is used because it blends with the screen and thus will not be visually distracting to the patient. Many perimetrists write directly on the screen with chalk, but this method is not recommended as it provides clues to the patient and can leave permanent marks on the screen. A gray artist's pencil leaves marks that the patient cannot see and are easily removed using a felt blackboard eraser.

Next plot several isopters kinetically, beginning with one that is located about 20° to 25° from fixation. Move the target along the meridians from the periphery toward the center and note (then mark) where the patient indicates that the target is seen. When testing near the vertical and horizontal meridians, do not test directly on the meridian, but rather a small distance to each side of these key lines. This will aid in the detection of nasal and vertical steps, because these meridians represent natural anatomical divisions in the visual pathway.

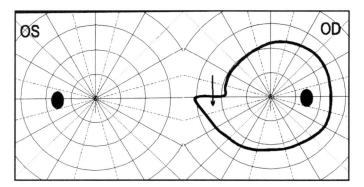

Figure 3-9. Confirming a superior nasal step. The stimulus is moved from the area of suspected nasal loss down across the horizontal meridian.

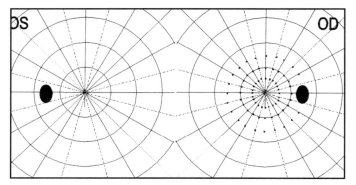

Figure 3-10. Typical test pattern of static testing on the tangent screen (OD).

When a nasal step is suspected, it can be confirmed as follows: place the test target in the area of suspected nasal loss and move it directly across the horizontal meridian. If it is seen as it crosses the meridian, the nasal step has been confirmed. Verify all vertical steps in a similar manner by testing across the vertical meridian. Figure 3-9 illustrates verifying a superior nasal step by moving the stimulus from the non-seeing area down across the horizontal meridian into an area where the patient had previously indicated that the stimulus could be seen.

If kinetic testing indicates that the patient doesn't have the extent of peripheral vision expected, further investigation is in order. If you double both the test size and the test distance, the isopter should double in its distance from fixation. "Tunnel" fields, where the isopter obtained from the more distant testing position overlaps or falls within the isopter obtained at the nearer testing position, is non-physiologic and a sign of malingering or non-organic visual loss.

After several isopters have been plotted, look for scotomas. This can be done using suprathreshold kinetic or static testing. For kinetic testing, move the target slowly along each meridian inside its isopter after instructing the patient to let you know if it disappears. Test for alertness by occasionally flipping the target over to expose the black side, thus making it disappear against the black screen. To test statistically, place the target in varying locations with the black side of the stimulus facing the patient, then turn it over to expose the target stimulus. Figure 3-10 shows a typical pattern for static presentations.

Scotoma should be mapped kinetically. Start by placing the target within the scotoma and then move it in some direction until it is seen. Mark that point. Return to your starting place within the scotoma and test again in a nearby direction. Continue testing in adjacent directions. As the shape of the scotoma becomes apparent, move the target perpendicular to its border to more accurately establish its size and shape. Once it has been characterized with one target, map it again in the same manner using a larger or smaller stimulus to get a measure of the steepness of the defect.

Recording the Results

Results are transcribed from the marked screen to polar charts using colored pencils or combinations of

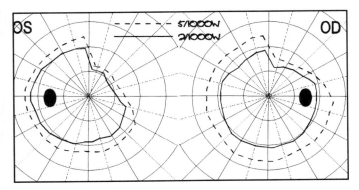

Figure 3-11. Example of tangent screen results.

light and heavy (or dashed and solid) lines. The isopters are labeled as to the target size and color and the testing distance. For example, if a white 2 mm test object is used on a 1 m tangent screen (1000 mm testing distance), the isopter obtained would be labeled "2/1000W." An example of a recording chart can be seen in Figure 3-11.

Results from static testing are indicated by small x's or dots at the positions of static presentations and labeled similarly.

Autoplot®

The Autoplot is a tangent screen system that employs a pantograph which projects light stimuli onto a specially designed gray tangent screen. The pantograph charts the results of the examination as it is performed. The size of the test stimuli can be changed quickly, and the stimuli can be turned on and off at will.

Goldmann Perimetry

- The Goldmann perimeter was designed to eliminate many of the factors leading to variability in visual field test results, to standardize visual field testing, and to minimize errors.

- Because of its unique design, the Goldmann perimeter is capable of performing both kinetic and static perimetry.

- Careful attention to pupil size, proper refractive correction, and testing technique can limit artifactual field loss.

- The intensity of the perimeter projector bulb should be calibrated at the beginning of the workday. The background illumination must be calibrated with the patient in place for the examination.

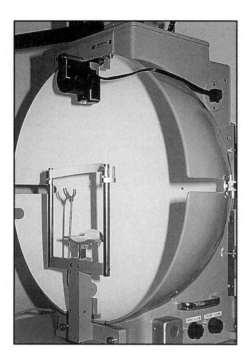

Figure 4-1. The Goldmann perimeter.

Introduction

Variability in manual perimetric techniques from one examiner to the next may lead to poor reproducibility of results, which in turn may lead to false conclusions regarding the progression of a patient's disease. Many factors (lighting irregularity, inaccurate distance, poor communication) may contribute to inconsistency and inaccuracy when performing tangent screen examinations. Another problem that arises with using a flat test surface is that, because the retina is curved, the test object presents a different size at different times as it is moved along the screen. Testing on a curved surface makes more sense. The Goldmann perimeter was designed to eliminate some of these factors in order to standardize visual field testing and minimize errors. Because of its unique design, the machine is capable of performing both kinetic and static perimetry. Ninety-five degrees on either side of fixation can be examined.

Machine Design

The Goldmann perimeter, illustrated in Figure 4-1, consists of a spherical bowl with a radius of curvature of 30 cm and a projector system capable of presenting a stimulus anywhere within the bowl. The bowl interior is painted matte white. The bowl is illuminated by a hooded lamp located at the top of the bowl. Light from this lamp is also projected through a movable hollow lever arm; this provides the stimulus, which is projected onto the bowl. Because the same lamp lights both the bowl and the stimulus, any variation in brightness affects the background and target equally. The projection arm is moved by means of a pantograph handle on the back of the perimeter. The pantograph is moved across a vertical chart holder. With a chart in place, the position of the pantograph corresponds to the stimulus position in the bowl. The right side of the instrument has a switch for turning the stimulus on and off. The stimulus is elliptical, and its size can be varied from 1/16 mm^2 up to 64 mm^2. The size and brightness of the stimulus is controlled by four levers. Stimulus color may be changed by using colored filters. The ratio of background to stimulus brightness is critical for accurate fields. However, this ratio can be disturbed by the reflectivity of the patient's skin and clothing. Thus the instrument must be calibrated before each exam with the patient in place at the perimeter.

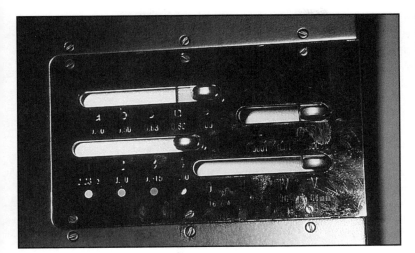

Figure 4-2. The stimulus control levers on the Goldmann perimeter.

There is a telescope in the back of the instrument to allow the examiner to continually view the patient's fixation. Patient position (up/down, left/right) is controlled by knobs on the back of the machine.

The Goldmann perimeter is designed to test the visual field with standardized background illumination (31.5 asb) and a projected target with a maximum intensity of 1000 asb. The target can be adjusted to six different sizes by means of diaphragms and to 60 intensity levels by means of grey filters. The background illumination is adjustable by a shutter and the maximum stimulus brightness by means of a rheostat. A light meter is provided to allow for the proper calibration of the instrument at the beginning of the examination. Examination conditions are held constant, and the visual fields recorded at various times under the same conditions can be compared over a period of years with minimal risk of error, enhancing the probability of detecting small changes in the field due to disease.

Basic Perimeter Operation

Stimulus Selection

The size and intensity of the test stimulus is set by means of four levers—one for the size and three for the intensity, as seen in Figure 4-2. These levers are located above the recording chart to the right of the fixation monitoring telescope. The stimulus size lever has six positions numbered 0, I, II, III, IV, and V, corresponding to 1/64, 1/4, 1, 4, 16, and 64 mm^2 respectively. A change in two places is the equivalent of a four-fold change in diameter and a 16-fold change in stimulus area, equivalent to a ten-fold (10 dB or one log unit) change in intensity. Thus, each step represents a 5 dB (0.5 log unit) change in intensity. The stimulus size I (with no intensity filters interposed) is the standard maximum stimulus and is equivalent to 1,000 asb in intensity. Intensity is decreased by changing to the stimulus size 0, representing a 5 dB attenuation (dimming). Increased intensity is simulated by switching to the larger stimulus sizes; the bulb cannot be made any brighter, but changing the size from the I to the V is equivalent to a 100-fold increase in intensity (two log units). The size 0 stimulus is rarely used.

The other three levers control the stimulus intensity. One lever has four positions, numbered 1 through 4. As the numbers decrease, the stimulus intensity decreases by 0.5 log units. Position 4 is unfiltered. Increasingly dense filters are interposed in front of the projected stimulus as the number decreases, up to a total of two log units of attenuation. The next lever has five positions labeled "a" through "e," and each stop decreases the stimulus by one dB, with "e" being unfiltered. By using combinations of lever positions, it is possible to step through the entire range of available stimulus intensities in one dB steps. The final lever, located in the upper right, has three positions. The position farthest to the right has no filter. The middle position, represented by a single bar, attenuates the stimulus intensity by two full log units. The two bar position is another two log units of attenuation. This lever is usually left in the fully open position to the right, unless very dim stimuli are required for determining foveal sensitivity.

The combination of the Roman numeral for stimulus size, and Arabic number and alphabet letter for stimulus intensity are combined to name the test stimulus and the corresponding isopter. For example, the standard stimulus is the stimulus size I with the filters fully off (equal to 1,000 asb), and would be represented as I_4e. A single or double bar over the alphabetical letter would indicate the position of the third bar lever. No bar is used if this lever is in the right hand position.

Table 4-1 shows the intensity values in asb for all of the available Goldmann stimuli. Note that there may be more than one way to obtain a given stimulus intensity. The relative dB scale is given in the table, with the reference (0 dB) being equal to 1,000 asb. Intensity levels greater than 1,000 asb are not available as the bulb cannot be made any brighter. However, the use of stimuli larger than the size I is the same in effect as using a brighter bulb.

Stimulus Control

The Goldmann perimeter has a shutter control that determines whether or not the stimulus is projected into the bowl. The knob is shown in Figure 4-3. The shutter control on some models is adjustable so the operator can determine whether the stimulus is seen when the shutter control lever is in the up or down position. Usually it is set so that the stimulus is projected when the lever is down and turned off when the lever is up. The lever moves silently so that the patient cannot respond to its noise. The shutter is used to turn the stimulus on and off for static testing. In this case, it is left off until the stimulus is positioned at the point to be tested, momentarily turned on to await a patient response, and the turned off for movement to the next position. It may also be left in the on position for kinetic testing. In kinetic testing, the stimulus is moved to the periphery of the meridian to be tested in an area expected to be non-seeing (or alternately within the center of a scotoma), turned on and left on, then moved toward expected seeing areas.

The position of the stimulus within the bowl is determined by the position of the pantograph handle as seen in Figure 4-4. The projection system (Figure 4-5) is designed so that the position of the handle on the recording chart corresponds to the position of the stimulus within the bowl. In other words, the stimulus will be projected to the area within the visual field of the eye being tested while the handle is over the same spot on the recording chart. The stimulus can be moved over the full surface of the bowl. By placing a pencil within the handle, the recording chart can be marked as soon as the patient reports that the stimulus has been seen, indicating that the isopter boundary has been crossed.

Basic Techniques for Stimulus Movement

One of the advantages of operator controlled (manual) perimetry as done with the Goldmann is the ability of the operator to customize the test to the patient's ability. As a general rule, when performing kinetic perimetry the stimulus should be moved at about 5° per second. Movement faster than this may result in isopters being mapped as smaller than they really are, because the patient may have seen the stimulus well before he or she could actually respond. Slower movement gives the patient time to find the stimulus by searching movements, and may result in false positive responses, making the field look larger (and better) than it really is. Move the stimulus steadily and only in one direction, do not oscillate it. The stimulus should always be moved from areas of non-seeing toward seeing areas because the patient can only signal when the stimulus is first seen, not when it disappears. This applies to mapping the blind spot, mapping the boundaries of isopters, and exploring the extent of scotomata detected by static stimulus presentations. Map the boundaries of isopters by randomly selecting the meridian in which to move the stimulus and do not follow a set pattern for selecting the next meridian. You don't want to give the patient an opportunity to predict where the next stimulus is coming from.

Table 4-1
Effective Decibel/Apostilb/Goldmann Equivalents

dB	Asb	0	I	II	III	IV	V
-20	100,000						V4e
-19	79,433						V4d
-18	63,096						V4c
-17	50,119						V4b
-16	39,811						V4a
-15	31,623					IV4e	V3e
-14	25,119					IV4d	V3d
-13	19,953					1V4c	V3c
-12	15,849					IV4b	V3b
-11	12,589					IV4a	V3a
-10	10,000				III4e	IV3e	V2e
-9	7,943				III4d	IV3d	V2d
-8	6,310				III4c	IV3c	V2c
-7	5,012				III4b	IV3b	V2b
-6	3,981				III4a	IV3a	V2a
-5	3,162			II4e	III3e	IV2e	V1e
-4	2,512			II4d	III3d	IV2d	V1d
-3	1,995			II4c	III3c	IV2c	V1c
-2	1,585			II4b	III3b	IV2b	V1b
-1	1,259			II4a	III3a	IV2a	V1a
0	1,000		I4e	II3e	III2e	IV1e	
1	794		I4d	II3d	III2d	IV1d	
2	631		I4c	II3c	III2c	IV1c	
3	501		I4b	II3d	III2b	IV1b	
4	398		I4a	II3a	III2a	IV1a	
5	316	04e	I3e	II2e	III1e		
6	251	04d	I3d	II2d	III1d		
7	200	04c	I3c	II2c	III1c		
8	158	04b	I3d	II2b	III1b		
9	126	04a	I3a	II2a	III1a		
10	100	03e	I2e	II1e			
11	79	03d	I2d	II1d			
12	63	03c	I2c	II1c			
13	50	03b	I2b	II1b			
14	40	03a	I2a	II1a			
15	32	02e	I1e				
16	25	02d	I1d				
17	20	02c	I1c				
18	16	02b	I1b				
19	13	02a	I1a				
20	10	01e					
21	8	01d					
22	6	01c					
23	5	01b					
24	3	01a					

Dimmer stimuli may be obtained by use of the "bar" lever. Each bar attenuates the stimulus by two log units.

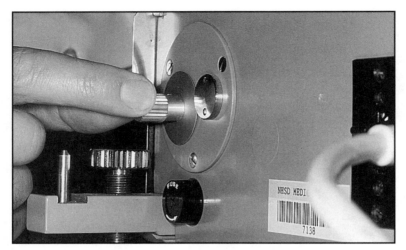

Figure 4-3. The shutter control knob. Pushing the knob down turns the stimulus on and releasing it will allow it to spring back to the off position. Rotating the knob 180° will reverse the switch; it will always be on unless the knob is pushed down to momentarily turn it off.

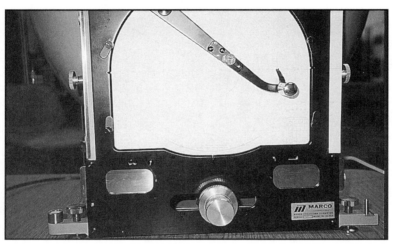

Figure 4-4. The pantograph (stimulus movement apparatus) control handle.

Technician Functions During a Test

In addition to selecting the stimuli, moving the stimuli, controlling the shutter, and recording the patient's responses, there are some other things the technician must do during a test. Fixation must be monitored through the telescope to make sure the patient is fixating steadily. Poor fixation behavior prevents the examiner from knowing where the stimulus was in the patient's visual field when the response button was pushed and leads to an incorrect map. It is possible for the examiner to monitor fixation with one eye while the other eye watches the location of the stimulus position control handle. (It takes practice.) Figure 4-6 illustrates the proper position for the technician with the right hand on the shutter control, the left hand on the pantograph handle (with a marking pencil in place), the left eye viewing the patient through the telescope, and the right eye looking at the recording chart.

Patients should be reinstructed as the test proceeds, particularly with regard to fixation behavior, and occasionally need to be reminded to push the button when the light is seen. It is a good idea to periodically project a larger, brighter stimulus within the boundary of an isopter mapped with a smaller, dimmer stimulus as a test of the patient's alertness. Failure to respond indicates a false negative response, and may indicate that the patient is inattentive. It is a good idea to set the shutter control so that the stimulus is *on* when the handle is depressed. This leaves both hands free for marking the stimulus position after the response button has been pressed.

Figure 4-5. Overview of the mechanism that moves the stimulus projector within the bowl as the handle is moved over the recording chart.

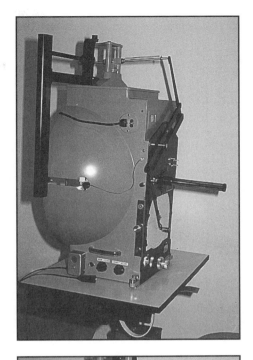

Figure 4-6. Examiner properly positioned to perform a test.

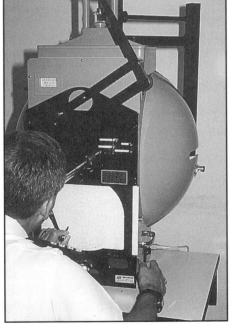

The Recording Chart

A blank Goldmann visual field recording chart is shown in Figure 4-7. Make sure the chart is properly positioned in its holder to ensure that the recorded points correspond to the position of the projected stimulus. The chart should be labeled with the patient's name and other identifying data, date of the examination, pupil size, distance refraction, and the near lens used for the central 30°. The visual acuity and diagnosis, if

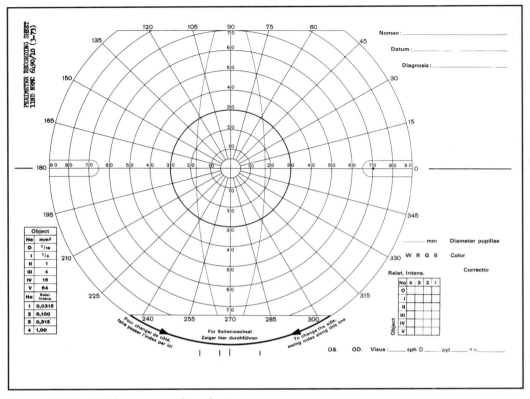

Figure 4-7. The Goldmann recording chart.

known, may also be listed. Each isopter should be recorded using a different colored pencil. The standard color coding of isopters is given in Table 4-2.

The lower right hand corner of the chart contains a relative intensity grid, which can be used to indicate the color used for each isopter. The isopters should also be individually labeled with the isopter name. Areas of scotomata should be labeled with the target that was *not* seen. Finally, comments regarding the patient's cooperation, fixation ability, and validity of responses should be made on the right side of the chart.

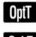

Testing a Patient

Prior to testing any patient, there are some general principles that should be followed. The location of the machine in the office or clinic is important. Testing should take place in an area free of distractions and extraneous noise. There should be no direct light falling on the bowl. Room light should be controlled with a dimmer. Finally, the visual field area should be free of foot traffic, doors or windows opening and closing, conversations, etc, so that the patient (and the examiner) can concentrate on the performance of the examination. Provide comfortable, adjustable chairs or stools for the patient, and make sure the machine is placed on a table that can be adjusted to fit the patient's height. Ensuring patient comfort and minimizing distractions will help to enhance performance and minimize errors.

Machine Preparation for an Examination

Place a blank recording chart into the holder, making sure to align the center marks for the horizontal and vertical meridia with the notches in the holder. Tighten the side clamps to prevent the paper from moving.

Table 4-2
Isopter Color Coding

Isopter Name	Color
I1e	yellow
I2e	red
I3e	green
I4e	blue
II4e	orange
III4e	purple
IV4e	brown
V4e	black

Calibrate the Stimulus Intensity

The Goldmann perimeter contains a light meter, which is used to make sure that the projector bulb is capable of generating at least a 1,000 asb stimulus. It may be located within the bowl or externally mounted, and either permanently attached or removable. It is necessary to make sure that the bulb is bright enough so that each isopter is of the correct intensity, thus maintaining the standardization of the test conditions. Calibration of the stimulus intensity must be performed at the beginning of each day.

To calibrate the projector bulb, first place the pantograph handle at the preset position found on the right side of the instrument (as the examiner faces the recording chart). The preset position is at 70° temporal to the fixation point for the right eye. There may be a hole into which a pin on the pantograph handle is inserted.

Next, position the light meter if it is not permanently mounted. Set the stimulus to V4e and move the small flag or occluder out of the light path, allowing the projected light to fall onto the light meter. Figure 4-8 shows the light meter on one Goldmann model.

Make sure the stimulus shutter is open. Adjust the intensity rheostat (Figure 4-9) until the light meter scale reads 1,000 asb (Figure 4-10). If 1,000 asb cannot be obtained, first try reversing the bulb in its socket or reversing the wire connecting the bulb to the power source. If that doesn't achieve the proper intensity, replace the bulb. Remove the light meter (if not built in) and place the meter in a drawer protected from light. Cover the light path with the occluder.

Correcting Lens

The bowl must be in focus for the patient to clearly see the projected stimuli. This requires the use of a correcting lens, determined from the distance refraction and an add based on the patient's age. The refractometric measurement should be recent and should yield visual acuity within two lines of the best acuity recorded in the patient's medical record. The visual acuity should be tested prior to beginning the visual field examination. If acuity is reduced (and perhaps improved with a pinhole), refractometry should be performed. Use the spherical equivalent if the cylindric correction is 1 diopter or less. (The spherical equivalent is determined by adding one half of the cylinder power to the spherical power.) Next, determine the add based on the patient's age and the perimeter bowl size. Remember that patients who have no accommodation (aphakic or pseudophakic patients, or anyone who has been dilated) require the maximum add, regardless of their age. Consult the user's manual for the machine; it should contain recommendations for the proper additions to be used.

Place the correcting lens into the holder provided inside the bowl (Figure 4-11). Make sure that the lenses are the "rimless" variety, (Figure 4-12); otherwise the thick black edge of the trial lens could cause artifactual loss. The lens must be positioned as close as possible to the eye being tested, but should not contact

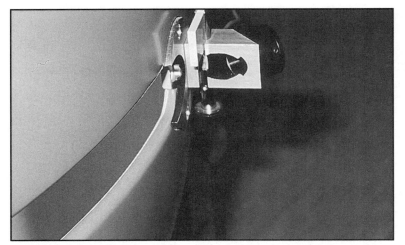

Figure 4-8. The light meter for calibrating the stimulus intensity. The white flag is in the "up" position to allow the projected V4e stimulus to fall on the light meter.

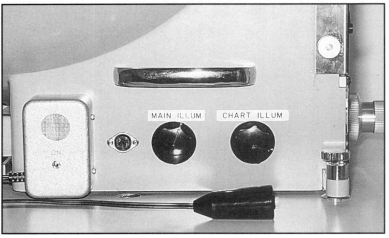

Figure 4-9. The rheostat for adjusting the stimulus intensity. Also shown is the adjustment knob for the back illumination of the recording chart and the patient response button.

the lashes. Also, be sure to remove the correcting lens and holder when testing outside the central 30°.

Further discussion of correcting lenses can be found in Chapter 5. A discussion of errors due to incorrect lens selection or placement is given in Chapter 7.

Patient Preparation

Pupils

Small pupils decrease the amount of light entering the eye and may result in patients missing stimuli that should be seen. The light needs to be made larger or brighter to elicit a response, giving the impression that the patient's sensitivity is reduced. This is particularly important in threshold perimetry, but in Goldmann perimetry the isopters will appear contracted relative to what they should be for a given patient. Media opacities, such as cataract, worsen the effect of miosis.

The critical size for the pupil is between 2 mm and 3 mm. Therefore, pupils less than 2 mm should be dilated for the visual field examination, unless it is not safe to do so. Remember that dilating the pupil will most likely affect the distance refraction. The refractometry must thus be checked after dilation. Because dilation eliminates the patient's ability to accommodate, the full add for the machine being used must be added to the new distance lens (usually +3.00).

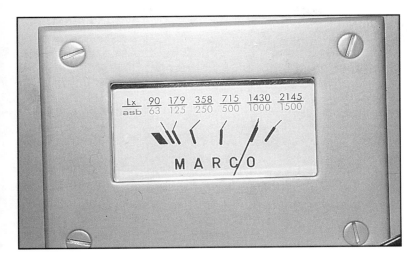

Figure 4-10. The light meter scale with the bulb properly adjusted to 1,000 asb.

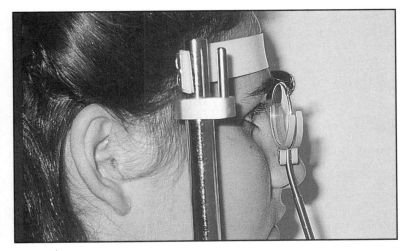

Figure 4-11. The correcting lens holder.

It may be convenient to schedule a dilated fundus exam on the same day as the visual field if the patient needs to be dilated for the field anyway. After dilation, the refractive measurement is checked and the fundus examined. The field is then performed. This also reduces the number of fields that must be repeated due to inadequate pupil size.

Whether or not the pupils require dilation, make sure to measure the pupil diameter using the millimeter reticle found in the fixation telescope. The reticule and the patient's eye will be visible in the telescope when the patient is properly positioned. Record the pupil size on the recording chart.

Lids and Brows

Drooping lids (ptosis) and/or brows may interfere with the patient's ability to see stimuli in the superior visual field, giving the appearance of a field loss that often resembles a glaucoma defect. Elevating the overhanging tissue with tape will often eliminate the artifactual defect. Be careful not to tape too high so as not to interfere with the patient's ability to blink.

Patient Instructions

Visual field testing can be difficult for the patient as well as the examiner. The best possible results will be obtained if the patient is aware of what is going to be done and why it is being done. An explanation of

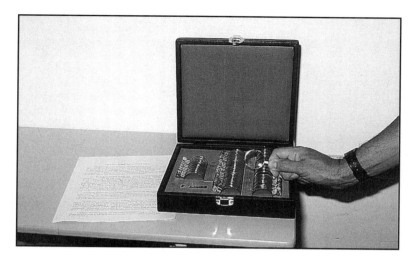

Figure 4-12. "Rim-less" correcting lenses best suited for visual field testing.

the testing procedures can alleviate anxiety and help the patient to perform better. The patient should be told about maintaining fixation on the center spot, that fixation will be monitored through the telescope, and that he or she should push the response button when the light is seen. The patient should also be encouraged to let the examiner know if the targets or the center spot are not in focus and if a rest period is needed.

What the Patient Needs to Know

- This is a test of your side or peripheral vision.

- We test one eye at a time so one eye will be covered.

- When we start the test, your chin will be in the cup and your forehead against this bar. Your job for the entire test is to look at this light here in the middle. As you look in the center, another light will come on somewhere inside the bowl. When you first think you see the light, press this button.

- You won't see the target light all the time. Sometimes you may seem to go for a long time without seeing anything. Don't worry; just be patient until the light appears again. The main thing is not to look for the light. Always look right here in the center.

- Don't wait for the light to get all the way to you. Press the button when you first think you see it. Any areas that seem inconsistent will be rechecked.

- I have a little telescope on the other side of the machine, and I can see your eye. If I notice that you are looking around instead of at the center, I'll remind you to look straight ahead.

- From time to time you'll feel your head move slightly as I keep your position adjusted.

- If you need to rest, let me know.

- Be sure not to stare. You can blink whenever you need to.

- If you are uncomfortable, let me know.

Patient instruction common to both Goldmann and automated perimetry is covered in detail in Chapter 5.

Patient Positioning

First, occlude the non-tested eye. (Usually the right eye is tested first.) If a white occluder is used, the covered eye will be maintained in a light adapted state, facilitating its testing later on. Next, position the patient in the machine. The machine height and/or the patient's chair should be adjusted so that the patient's forehead can comfortably rest against the headrest when the chin is in the chinrest. Adjust the chinrest up, down, left, and right until the eye is visible in the telescope and centered in the reticle. The pupil size may now be measured and recorded.

Calibrate the Intensity of the Background Illumination

Because patients' skin tone and clothing reflect varying amounts of light into the bowl, the background illumination must be calibrated for each patient. To perform this calibration, set the projector arm to the position used for calibrating the bulb (the bulb should already be adjusted to 1,000 asb). Make sure the cover is over the light path. Set the stimulus to V1e (the combination of the "1" and the "e" filters dims the stimulus to 31.5 asb). Position the patient in the instrument. Look into the bowl from the left side toward the target on the right. Adjust the knob that controls the background illumination until the brightness of the target's center and periphery are of equal intensity. On one model this is accomplished by raising or lowering a hood on the bulb housing (Figure 4-13). This adjustment, done by visual comparison, is more accurate than using a light meter. This calibration is critical to maintaining reproducibility of visual fields over time. Remember to do this calibration with each patient *and* with the patient in position at the perimeter. Consult the manufacturer's manual for the proper calibration method for your machine.

Test Strategies

There are as many ways to conduct a visual field examination with the Goldmann perimeter as there are examiners. Adopting some sort of standard technique helps to increase reproducibility of the exam findings. The significance of reproducibility is that if a follow-up field shows apparent worsening, it is more likely to be due to the underlying disease process than due to a variation in technique. The technique described below is excellent for visual field testing of glaucoma patients. It was developed by Drs. Armaly and Drance and is known as the Armaly/Drance screening protocol. Performed properly, it will elicit up to 90% of early glaucoma defects and will take 12 minutes or less in an eye with few defects. Refer to Figure 4-14, which summarizes the Armaly/Drance protocol, as the various techniques are described. Although the Armaly/Drance screening was intended for glaucoma, similar techniques can be employed for patients with suspected or known neurological disease; the main difference is in the meridian explored for steps (horizontal for glaucoma, vertical for neurological).

Screening

The selection of a test strategy is usually determined by the patient's diagnosis or suspected disease. Patients with glaucoma should be tested with attention to the nasal areas and the horizontal midline, because this is where defects are most likely to occur. Particular attention must be paid to the central 30°, with static searches to detect isolated scotomata (technique follows). Patients with suspected neurological disease must be carefully tested for asymmetrical loss across the vertical midline. Remember that the correcting lens is necessary for the central 30°, but should be removed for testing the periphery.

Screening the visual field with the Goldmann perimeter is defined in a different sense than screening with an automated threshold perimeter. In automated perimetry, as discussed in the next chapter, screening implies a quick method of testing a number of points relative to known normal threshold values and determining whether or not the patient is "normal" at each point. The result is usually displayed as an array of

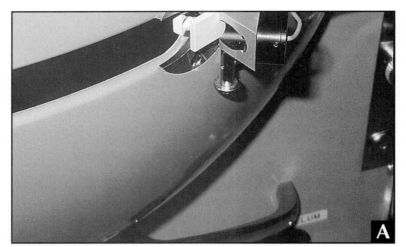

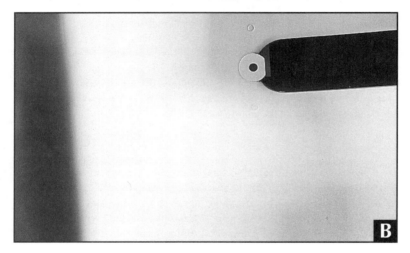

Figure 4-13. Adjusting the background illumination. (A) The flag is "down," covering the light meter. (B) View of the target. The projected stimulus (V1e) will be reflected off the white flag as the light passes through the opening in the target.

symbols indicating which points are presumed to be normal and which are not. The island of vision is not precisely mapped. Screening on the Goldmann, on the other hand, implies that a map of the island of vision will be drawn in isopter format, with no comparison to "normal." It also implies that the entire visual field has not been tested, which would be technically difficult and time-consuming; instead, the visual field is rapidly screened for defects.

Central Isopters

With the proper correcting lens in place, begin the test by determining the initial stimulus in an area approximately 25° in the temporal field (to the patient's right for a right eye and to the left for a left eye) as shown in Figure 4-14, top left. Make sure the shutter is off, set the stimulus to I1e, pick a spot 5° above or below the horizontal midline, check fixation, and briefly open the shutter by depressing the lever. The stimulus should be on for no more than approximately 0.2 seconds. (See how long that is by using a stopwatch prior to testing a patient; don't attempt to time each stimulus.) Step through the stimulus intensities and sizes, making the stimulus larger or brighter in 5 dB steps (Roman numerals or Arabic numerals) in response to the patient's responses. If the I1e is not seen, for example, try the I2e or III1e. Keep increasing the stimulus in 5 dB steps until you find a stimulus to which the patient reliably and consistently responds. If the I1e is seen, decrease the stimulus in 5 dB steps until the stimulus is not seen, the initial stimulus will then be the previous one used prior to the non-response.

Next, use this initial stimulus to map the blind spot. The blind spot is located at approximately 15° tem-

(C) The hood is moved up and down (changing the background illumination) until the edge of the target (illuminated by the background) matches the light seen in the center of the ring (the projected V1e stimulus reflected off the white flag). Because the center light is 31.5 asb, the background will similarly be 31.5 asb when a match is obtained.

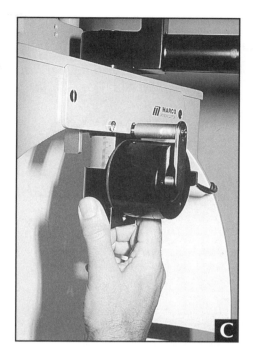

poral to fixation, slightly below the horizontal midline. Move the projector to this area and briefly expose the stimulus. There should be no response. Beginning at the spot where there is no response, open the shutter, leave it open, and move the stimulus outward in any direction until the patient responds. Mark that point. Return to the non-seen area and move in another direction until seen. Four or five presentations should be sufficient to map the blind spot, but you can be more precise if you use all eight "cardinal" directions (up, down, left, right, and each position in between).

The next step, still using the initial stimulus, is to map a central isopter. Move the projector to about 40° to 50° from the center along a meridian not located on the horizontal or vertical midline. (Usually, the meridia used are multiples of 30°.) Check fixation, turn on the stimulus (and leave it on), and slowly move along the meridian (5° per second) toward fixation. Record the point at which the patient responds, indicating that the stimulus has crossed from non-seeing to seeing. Repeat for each meridian, choosing the next one at random, until you have tested at 30°, 60°, 120°, 150°, 210°, 240°, 300°, and 330° (Figure 4-14, bottom left). Next, repeat this kinetic testing at each 5° meridian on either side of the four midlines (superior vertical, inferior vertical, temporal horizontal, and nasal horizontal). This technique will help to localize "steps" across the midline, indicating disease. The normal isopter shape is a somewhat horizontally oval, wider in the temporal field than elsewhere. Any apparent constrictions in the field to the initial isopter should be explored with a larger (or brighter) and smaller (or dimmer) test object.

Verify or Specifically Look for Steps

Steps may be easily verified by moving the stimulus perpendicularly across the meridian from the non-seeing area toward the midline (Figure 4-14, top right). If a true step is present, the patient will respond as soon as the midline is crossed. Searches can be done by presenting paired static stimuli on either side of the midline within 5° to 10° of the isopter boundary using sequentially smaller or dimmer stimuli. Confirm such steps by the kinetic method described above. Concentrate on the appropriate meridian for the patient's disease process—vertical for neurological disease, horizontal for glaucoma or other optic neuropathy.

Test the Peripheral Field

Now test outside the central 30°. Remove the correcting lens. Then determine the initial stimulus at a point 40° to 50° temporal to fixation, 5° above or below the horizontal midline (in the same manner as that used to

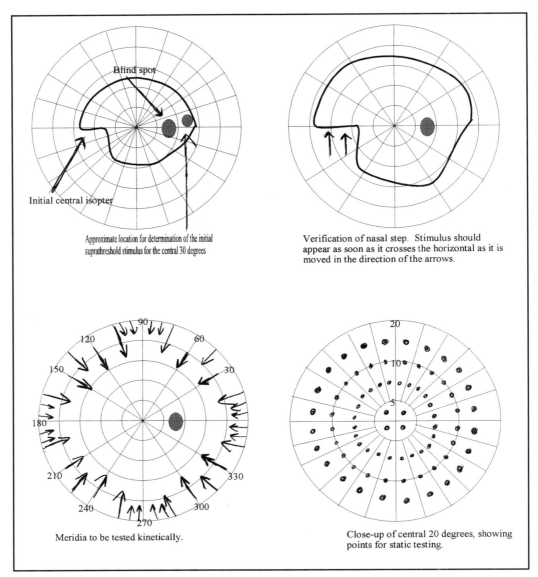

Figure 4-14. The Armaly/Drance screening technique. Top left, location of test point for initial stimulus, blindspot, and initial central isopter. Bottom left, meridia for kinetic testing. Top right, verification of nasal step. Bottom right, points for static testing within the central 20°.

determine the initial stimulus for central testing) beginning with the I2e. If any defects are seen, map an additional one or two isopters with brighter (or larger) or dimmer (or smaller) stimuli. Verify any identified steps.

Some examiners will begin the examination with no correcting lens, testing outside of the central 30° first, kinetically as described above and statically as described below. The correcting lens is then placed, and the center field is tested. The order of the examination is not that important, but both the center and the periphery should be tested.

Static Search for Central Scotomata

As the stimulus is moved centrally along each meridian, the boundary is marked as the stimulus passes from areas of non-seeing into seeing areas. However, it is quite possible to have areas of decreased sensitivity within the boundary mapped by the kinetic technique. The examiner could conceivably discover these areas by continuing to move the stimulus centrally after the isopter boundary has been crossed and ask the patient to respond if and when the stimulus disappears. However, this technique would often fail to detect such central scotomata, because once the patient becomes aware of the presence of the stimulus, he or she becomes attentive to it, and may not be able to tell if it enters a new area of non-seeing. For this reason, central scotomata should be searched for by a static stimulus presentation technique.

To test statically, use the stimulus corresponding to the largest isopter within the central 30°. Make sure the correcting lens is in place. Turn the stimulus off and move the projector to the point to be tested. The areas to be covered include points at the center of each 2.5° quadrant and along each 15° meridian at 5°, 10°, and 15° above and below the horizontal midline (Figure 4-14, bottom right). This covers the Bjerrum area, where early paracentral defects are likely to occur. Present the stimulus at each point by turning the stimulus on for approximately 0.2 seconds, turning it off, and noting the patient's response. Seen points can be marked with a dot and missed points with an X. Finally, explore each missed point kinetically, moving from the missed point outward in each cardinal direction. This will define the full extent of the scotoma.

Threshold (Static) Perimetry with the Goldmann Perimeter

The Goldmann perimeter may be set up to statically define threshold along a single meridian and generate a profile cut through the island of vision. The machine must be equipped with a special static projection device and an intensity ruler. Testing at each point is done by beginning with a stimulus that is too small or too dim to be seen (infrathreshold) and varying the intensity in 1 dB steps until it is seen. Measurements are made every 3° to 5° along the meridian, and every 1° to 2° in areas in which depression (ie, less than normal expected sensitivity) is found. Remember to use appropriate spectacle correction within the central 30°.

Static threshold testing with the Goldmann perimeter has largely been replaced by automated perimetry in which threshold testing may be carried out at each point in the test grid. The reader is referred to the owner's manual for a complete description of setting up the machine for this test and referred to other texts for a more complete description of the technique.

A Checklist for Goldmann Perimetry

1. Turn machine on and calibrate the stimulus intensity (once daily).
2. Position the recording chart.
3. Select the correcting lens according to the patient's distance refractometric measurement, combine with appropriate add power, and place in the lens holder.
4. Instruct the patient as to the test procedures.
5. Occlude the non-tested eye and position the patient comfortably at the machine. Position the correcting lens as close to the eye as possible without touching the lashes.
6. Calibrate the background illumination.
7. Adjust the focus on the telescope so that the patient's eye is clearly seen. Note the pupil size.
8. Using static techniques, determine the suprathreshold stimulus intensity at a point approximately 25° temporal to fixation, slightly above or below the horizontal.
9. Using this stimulus, kinetically map the blind spot and a central isopter.
10. Perform static searches within the arcuate areas for scotomata.

11. Map two additional kinetic isopters, one larger and one smaller than the initial.
12. Verify all steps.
13. Kinetically explore all missed static presentations to map any scotomata.
14. Remove the correcting lens, determine a peripheral suprathreshold stimulus statically at 50°, and map two to three peripheral isopters, verifying steps.
15. Make sure all necessary information has been recorded on the chart.
16. Test the fellow eye.

Automated Perimetry

- Automated visual field testing systems have been developed in an attempt to eliminate some of the difficulties of manual perimetry.

- The system used to perform visual field testing should be organized in such a way as to minimize impediments to satisfactory perimetry and to maximize the capabilities of the machine.

- Useful results from automated perimetry depend heavily on communication among all of the parties concerned—the health care provider, the technician, and the patient.

- Although most automated perimeters are capable of performing both suprathreshold screening and threshold tests, the most useful information is obtained with full threshold tests.

Rationale for Automation in Perimetry

It should be obvious from the discussion of manual perimetry, particularly as performed with the Goldmann perimeter, that it is a difficult task. Administering a visual field test by Goldmann perimetry in a glaucoma patient, for example, requires a combination of kinetic (to define isopter boundaries) and static (to find nasal steps and paracentral defects) techniques, taking 20 to 30 minutes per eye. In addition, it may be difficult for a human examiner to avoid introducing bias into an otherwise subjective examination, thereby reducing the accuracy of the examination. An examiner may wish, consciously or unconsciously, for an examination to be "normal" and may fail to detect defects; similarly, nonexistent "defects" may be discovered if the examiner wishes them to be present. Follow-up examinations likewise become subject to inaccuracies, particularly if performed by different examiners, due to variations in technique as well as other "human" factors. Results of such examinations are also dependent on the interaction between the examiner (technician) and the patient and may be influenced by that interaction even in the absence of any visual field abnormalities.

Automated visual field testing systems have been developed in an attempt to eliminate some of the above problems. Computer controlled test procedures can be standardized and are not subject to examiner bias. In addition, visual field data can be manipulated by the computer into various formats that ease interpretation for the clinician. The data can also be stored, compared to known normals, and recalled at the time of follow-up procedures for evaluation. Finally, automation has allowed a transition from manually controlled (ie, by the technician) kinetic perimetry to computer controlled static threshold perimetry, which has been shown to detect loss (particularly centrally) earlier than the older techniques.

Various machine designs have evolved since the advent of perimetry automation. All machines perform static perimetry in one form or another, with most having the capability of determining threshold at the points tested. Some have the capacity to perform automated kinetic perimetry and define isopters. Stimulus presentation methods also vary. Some machines use the computer solely to control the test while other machines use either an internal or external computer for data storage and manipulation.

Machines and Manufacturers

The major brands of perimeters available today are from Zeiss-Humphrey (the Humphrey Field Analyzer), Interzeag (Octopus™), Dicon (TKS 4000™), and others (Marco, Bausch and Lomb). The reader is referred to the manufacturer's user's manual for complete information about the machine he or she is using. The discussion of automated perimetry that follows is intended to be applicable to most office situations, but because of the diversity of today's machines cannot be complete about any one instrument. The authors have the most experience with the Humphrey Field Analyzer, and the examples used in the remainder of the discussion will be from that machine.

Organizing a System for Automated Perimetry

Having an automated perimeter with all of its capabilities is not sufficient to guarantee optimal visual field testing. Taking advantage of all the machine has to offer requires an integrated system for management of visual field information—ordering it, obtaining it, printing it, storing it, retrieving it, interpreting it, and using it in patient care. The system used in your practice to perform visual field testing should be organized in such a way as to minimize impediments to satisfactory perimetry and to maximize the capabilities of the machine.

Figure 5-1. Visual field room with Humphrey Field Analyzer.

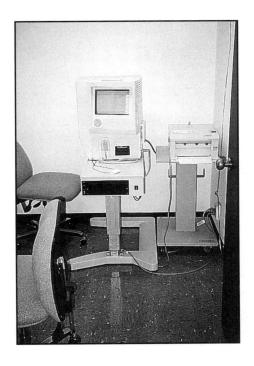

Machine Location

Automated perimetry is inherently difficult to perform comfortably and reliably. Tests are often long and tiring, and patients can easily become distracted, bored, or hypnotized. Therefore, the machine must be located in a place that is relatively free of noise or other sources of distraction. Preferably it should be housed in its own room, which should have adequate ventilation and be of comfortable temperature. The testing room must be big enough to hold the machine, patients of varying size and shape, the technician, and comfortable chairs for the patient and the technician. There should also be storage facilities for floppy disks, printer ribbons, and paper. The room lights should be on a dimmer switch to match the ambient lighting to that required for the machine being used. For example, some perimeters operate at a low background illumination, and the room lights should therefore be dimmed prior to beginning the test to allow the patient to become dark adapted. Other machines, such as the Humphrey Field Analyzer, operate under "photopic" conditions with a fairly bright background and do not require dark adaptation. The machine should be positioned so as to avoid stray light on the bowl, not only from any overhead lights but also from windows and doors, because any stray light may interfere with the patient's ability to detect the projected stimuli. The patient may respond to stray light thinking it is a projected stimulus, leading to false positive responses. Above all else, the patient's comfort and ability to concentrate on the task at hand are the main considerations in selecting a location for the machine.

Figure 5-1 is a photograph of a perimetry room containing a Humphrey Field Analyzer. The room is 6 ft wide and 8 ft long with the perimeter placed midway down the long wall on one side. The chairs are adjustable; adjusting the perimeter table and the patient chair ensures that a patient can be positioned comfortably at the machine. Not seen in the photo is a small desk. Trial lenses and the floppy disks for storage of patient data are placed on the table. In the drawers are extra floppy disks, paper, printer ribbons, and other supplies. The lights are installed with dimmer switches, which allow the room to be darkened sufficiently for the exam without making it difficult for the technician to find supplies. Prompts for the technician or instructions for the patient can be placed on the walls in the room. Figure 5-2 is a poster explaining fixation technique during foveal threshold determination. The poster serves as a reminder for the perimetrist in prompting the patient during the various initial stages of a test.

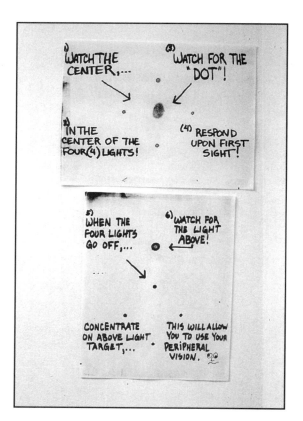

Figure 5-2. Example of technician "prompts" taped to a wall of examination room.

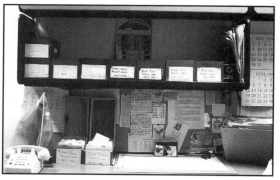

Figure 5-3. Technician desk area in dedicated perimetry space.

OptA   Technician Space

The technician needs a place for recording and filing patient data, storing the perimeter manual for ready reference, and locating old visual fields stored on disk. In a practice where many visual fields are performed, or where multiple machines may be in use at one time, it may be desirable to dedicate space for the technician outside the perimetry room. In practices where fewer fields are performed, the technician can make use of space in the perimetry room. Figure 5-3 shows the technician desk in the authors' clinic.

The boxes hold 3x5 visual field locator cards, which will be described in detail later in this chapter. The fan folder on the right holds visual field request forms for patients with appointments for visual field testing. The request forms contain information the technician needs in order to perform the exam, including the type of test, strategy, and printout desired, the patient's refractometric and phakic status, and follow-up information. The data needed by the technician to perform the test properly is discussed later in this chapter.

Figure 5-4. Patient instruction sheets (see also Table 5-4) conveniently placed outside of the visual field area, readily accessible for the patients.

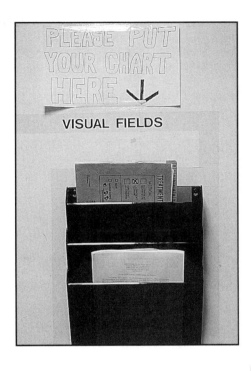

Patient Information
OptA

Useful results from automated perimetry depend heavily on communication among all of the parties concerned—the health care provider (the person who needs the information generated by the test), the technician (who has to administer the test and report the results back to the provider), and the patient (who must be informed about what is expected and be capable of performing properly). This communication loop goes from clinician to perimetrist to ensure the correct test performed properly, and from perimetrist to clinician as feedback on patient performance. There must be a flow of information from the provider to the technician, technician to patient, patient to machine, and ultimately all back to the provider. The location of the machine, the set-up of the system, and the operating procedures employed are all key components to be considered in order to obtain meaningful test results.

Obtaining interpretable results with automated perimetry may be enhanced when the patient understands what is being done and why. The patient should be given a brief explanation about the nature of the test and about what to expect during the examination. Performance can be enhanced by providing the arriving visual field patient with a handout explaining the exam. Figure 5-4 shows how patient handouts can be made available in the visual field waiting area, as in the authors' clinic. The medical record is placed in the box and the patient takes one of the information handouts. The patient then has the opportunity to read the handout while the technician is setting up for the examination. The contents of the handout will be discussed in detail later in this section.

Patient Data Storage and Retrieval
OptA

Some automated perimeters have the capability of storing test results. For example, visual fields are stored digitally on magnetic media with the Humphrey perimeter. Large amounts of data can thus be stored in a relatively small amount of space. (Two hundred visual field exams can fit on one 5¼-in floppy disk used by one Humphrey model.) Other machines use 3½-in floppy disks, dedicated hard drives, or external computers for storage. While this type of storage is highly reliable, data can be lost. Disk head crashes, accidental exposure to magnetic fields, and faulty diskettes, while not common occurrences, can lead to loss of

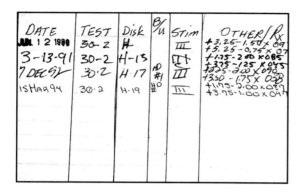

Figure 5-5. Back side of index card from patient visual field database.

visual fields. For this reason, multiple copies and frequent backing up of visual field data is vital. The recommended method of maintaining duplicate visual field data depends on the perimeter hardware. Follow the recommendations of the manufacturer.

Patient Visual Field Database

One of the greatest advantages of computerized perimetry is having quantitative data that the appropriate software can analyze for changes over time. An additional benefit on some machines is the ability to shorten testing procedures by using prior results as a starting point. However, in order to accomplish these things, the software must have access to the patient's previous examinations. If you are using an external floppy disk storage system, you have to be able to locate the disks containing the earlier data; if you are using more than one perimeter with hard drives, you must know which machine contains the desired fields. Thus, it is imperative to establish some sort of database. The essential information in the database should include the patient's name, test performed, stimulus size used, refractometric measurement used, and most importantly, which disks contain the patient's data. A well-organized system would allow follow-up testing even in the absence of the printout from the prior tests and/or without the medical record.

How you organize your system will depend on how big you expect your perimetry system to be and what type of information management system you use. For smaller practices, you may wish to make an entry in the patient's medical record indicating where the results of the visual fields are stored or write the information directly on the printout of the field.

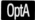 ### Card System

We have found an index card system to be useful and simple. A 3x5-in index card is filled out for each patient undergoing visual field testing. One side of the card contains identifying data, including name, social security number, date of birth, address, and telephone number. On the other side an entry is made for each examination, including the test performed, the date of the exam, stimulus size used, the refractometric measurement used, and the data storage disk(s) identification (Figure 5-5). When the patient returns for a follow-up examination, the card is pulled and the appropriate disk(s) located.

Computerized Relational Database

An alternative to keeping a card file is to place the database on an office or personal computer. Any database program, such as DBASE III+® (Ashton-Tate, 1985, 1986) or Microsoft Access®, can be used. A computer database is much like a card file. Each record in a database is like a single card in the card file, with each field in the database corresponding to an entry on the card. Computer databases are generally referred to as "flat" or "relational." Using the card file analogy, a flat database contains records where each card represents a single visual field examination. Patients with multiple visual field examinations would have multiple cards in the card file. In a relational database, information such as a patient's name and phone number would be stored only once; records with the patient's demographic data would include a unique value (a patient identification number) that would be related to records containing visual field data, such as what test was performed, when it was performed, and on what disk the field can be found. Using relational databases allows more flexibility in the design of the database and in later modifications, but either type can satisfy the needs for visual field record keeping.

Whatever type of database structure is used, the basic information required is the same as on the card file system described above. The advantage of a computerized database is that information can be located easily. This can provide a means for quality improvement in a practice and can be used in outcome analysis. For example, a practitioner might want to determine if the information obtained from central 30-2 threshold tests was any more useful in his practice than that from central 24-2 exams. The database could be queried to list the most recent 30 of each of those types of visual fields. The fields could be printed out and the comparison made. It is easy to add additional database fields of interest. For example, a field (here the word "field" refers to a line item on the data entry) could be added to indicate progression of visual field defects (improved, stable, or worse). The database could be queried to find all fields showing deterioration in a group of glaucoma patients and that information used to evaluate the effectiveness of therapy. There are a number of commercially available database software programs; selection of a program, designing the visual field database, and implementing its use is beyond the scope of this text and is left to the individual practice.

Testing the Patient

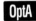

Test Selection

Most automated perimeters offer a wide variety of tests. Usually, the test to be performed is determined by the physician who ordered the test, but occasionally the decision is left to the technician. Therefore it is essential that the operator understand the capabilities of the machine being used. Once again, there is no substitution for thoroughly reading the manufacturer's manual. If there is any doubt about what information is desired, the decision should be left to the clinician.

Screening Tests

The majority of automated perimeters are capable of performing two different types of tests. Screening tests can be used for a quick assessment as to the presence or absence of visual field abnormalities. Using expected normal sensitivity values, points in the visual field are tested with values slightly brighter than should be necessary to elicit a response. This is known as "suprathreshold" testing. If the sensitivity is normal at a test point, the patient should respond. Lack of response is considered abnormal sensitivity for that point. Different strategies are usually available to characterize the nature of the abnormalities. Screening tests are designed to quickly tell whether or not a field is normal without actually drawing the map. Numerical data is not obtained, and there is no estimation of fluctuation. Also, because the individualized island of vision model is used to generate expected normals, small defects will be missed in a field with thresholds that all lie above the age corrected normals. Suppose that a patient has a 5 dB defect at a few field points, yet his entire hill of vision is otherwise 5 dB above the level expected for his age. A screening test comparing the shape of his island of vision using only stimuli 6 dB above expected (for shape) would miss the 5 dB local loss. A patient with an abnormal screening test requires further testing to delineate the nature of the abnormalities.

Figure 5-6 is a schematic of suprathreshold screening. For this figure, the lower numbers on the vertical axis represent brighter stimuli (lower dB numbers = less dimming of the maximum stimulus). Each point is tested with a stimulus 6 dB brighter than normally expected as depicted on the middle curve. At any point in the field where the 6 dB line lies below the patient's island of vision profile, the stimulus will be bright enough to elicit a response; if the test stimulus is above the island of vision profile it will be too dim to elicit a response. Thus, no responses will be obtained in the area of the scotoma centered around -10°. This portion of the field will be labeled as abnormal, but the actual shape of the island in this region has not been determined.

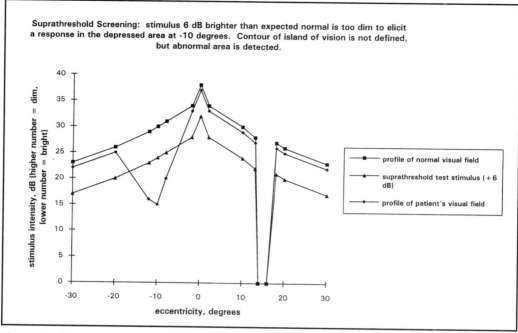

Figure 5-6. Theory underlying screening tests on automated perimeters.

Screening with Multiple Simultaneous Stimulus Presentations

Because screening methods are designed to detect abnormalities in the visual system, it would make sense that some sort of visual field test be incorporated into all eye examinations. Various methods have been developed in an attempt to provide adequate screening. Confrontation testing remains the mainstay for screening today, but is not sensitive enough to detect subtle visual field defects.

Dr. David O. Harrington, in conjunction with Dr. Milton Flocks, designed an instrument to rapidly screen the visual field through the use of simultaneously projected multiple stimuli. The device, known as the Harrington-Flocks screener, is depicted in Figure 5-7. The patient is in position for an examination with one eye occluded and the other fixating on a central dot. The examiner's finger is on the button, which will illuminate the dot pattern. The device projects a series of 10 patterns of dots and crosses to each eye, stimulating various portions of the visual field simultaneously. The dots, ranging in size from 1 mm near the center to 8 mm in the periphery, are printed in white fluorescent sulfide ink on a white background and are not visible in ordinary light. They become visible when illuminated with a flash of ultraviolet (black) light of 0.25 seconds duration (long enough to be seen but too short for a shift in fixation). Figure 5-8 illustrates the 10 patterns for the right eye. A mirror image set of 10 patterns is provided for the left eye, although presented in a different sequence.

Figure 5-9 illustrates the composite area of visual field covered by the 20 cards. As each card is exposed, the patient describes the pattern. If there is a defect in the visual field, the pattern will be described incorrectly. The most rapid screening is obtained when the patient simply reports how many dots were obtained, and, if the number is incorrect, then describes the pattern. A recording chart is used to mark the missed points, as depicted in Figure 5-10.

The series of cards and patterns covers most areas within the central 25°. The small cross on one card for each eye corresponds to the normal blind spot and should not be seen by someone with normal fixation behavior. The large cross on another card will be missed by someone with an "enlarged" blind spot. Figure 5-10 is an example of a defect found with the Harrington-Flocks screener. The pattern of missed points

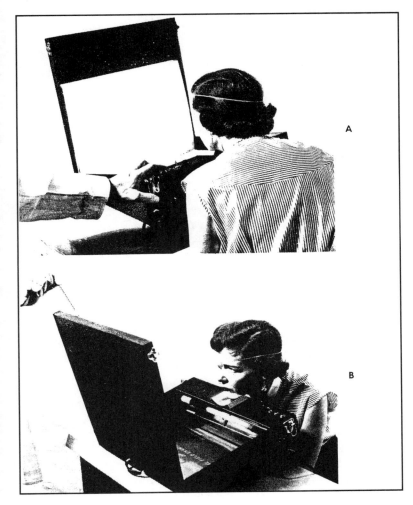

Figure 5-7. The Harrington-Flocks screener.

appears to represent a right-sided incongruous homonymous hemianopia. This defect was verified by tangent screen testing, illustrated in the bottom of the figure.

Simultaneous multiple stimulus screening was incorporated in an automated perimeter, the Dicon TKS 4000™. This machine uses a series of fixed light emitting diodes (LEDs) and a moving fixation device that the patient follows. Up to four stimuli, covering different areas of the visual field (depending on where the machine has "moved" the eye), may be exposed simultaneously. The patient indicates how many lights were seen by pushing the response button once for each stimulus, or by speaking the number into a small microphone incorporated near the headrest. (The machine may be programmed to recognize almost any language.) If the number is incorrect, the machine will test all of the points in that particular pattern until it determines the missed points. The field may be rapidly screened in under 5 minutes per eye.

Measuring the Visual Field

Threshold tests actually measure sensitivity at each test point to construct a map of the island of vision. Fluctuation measurements can be made and the numerical data generated can be stored and recalled for analysis with regard to change over time. Population-based normal values can be used for analytical purposes. It is recommended that threshold tests be used whenever possible in order to maximize the information obtained and minimize the need for retesting. Figure 5-11 illustrates how threshold testing can define the contour of the patient's island of vision.

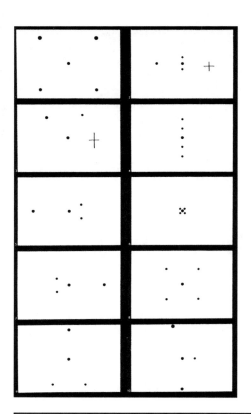

Figure 5-8. Patterns of dots presented to the right eye using the Harrington-Flocks screener.

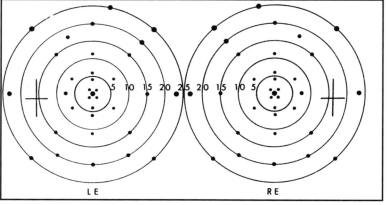

Figure 5-9. Composite area of visual field covered by the Harrington-Flocks screener.

Guidelines for Test Selection

It is recommended that the clinician review the available tests and strategies for the machine being used and set up a user defined menu (if that is an option) to meet the needs of the particular practice setting. Most practitioners will find four or five examination options will apply to the vast majority of clinical situations. Table 5-1 lists the types of patients commonly encountered in clinical practice and makes recommendations for appropriate tests from those available on the Humphrey Field Analyzer.

Note that "routine" visual field testing is not recommended. That would be like ordering neuro-imaging for everyone with a headache—the yield of pathologic results would be too low to justify the cost. Visual field testing should be used as an adjunctive test for the diagnosis and management of conditions known to affect the visual field and not as part of the routine eye examination of the patient with no relevant complaints.

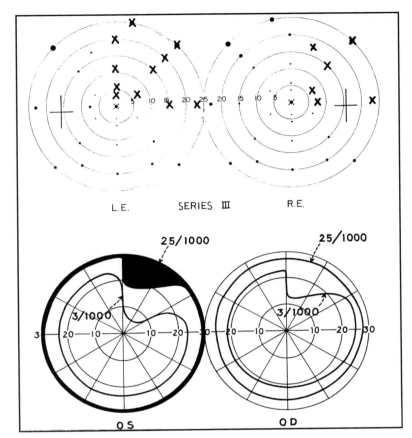

Figure 5-10. Recording chart for results from the Harrington-Flocks screener.

If a screening test is to be used, remember that the information obtained is limited. For example, the field shown in Figure 5-12 is useless clinically. The black squares symbolize points at which the patient did not push the response button when a brighter than expected normal stimulus was projected at the test point ("threshold related screen"). The few nasal misses and the two in the temporal field do not give the clinician any information on which to base a diagnosis. This patient must be tested again with a more quantitative test.

Figure 5-13 is an example of a threshold-related screen obtained from an elderly woman with limited capacity for the test procedures. Most of the points in the superior hemifield were missed at 6 dB brighter than expected normal. The pattern is suggestive of a superior altitudinal defect. It can be inferred that this is a very disturbed field, because the patient required a large stimulus and the central reference level was 30 dB. Still, it is not known what the magnitude of the loss is in the superior field: it could be anywhere from 7 dB up to absolute.

Additional information can be obtained by using the "three zone" strategy, as illustrated in Figure 5-14. Here, points not seen at 6 dB brighter than expected are tested with the maximum stimulus intensity. Points perceiving the maximum stimulus are labeled with the "X" indicating that they are relative defects while those not seen at 10,000 asb are labeled with the black square. The magnitude of the relative defects is not known. Worsening of the field over time can only be detected if the number of absolute defects increases at the expense of the relative defects. Therefore, if a screening test is to be used to follow a patient's course, it is recommended that a "quantify defects" strategy be used.

An example of a screening test performed with the quantify defects strategy is given in Figure 5-15. Here, threshold is determined for each point missed on the initial screen, and the printout shows the difference between the measured threshold and the expected value. The resultant defect depths can be followed

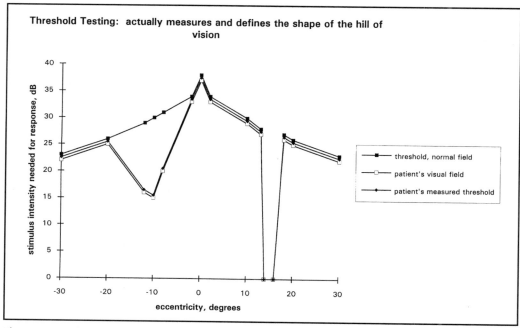

Figure 5-11. Theory underlying threshold tests on automated perimeters. Threshold tests draw the "map" of the island of vision.

over time. Although not as good as a threshold test, at least the quantify defects strategy of a screen offers some useful information. Whenever possible, it is desirable to follow patients with full threshold visual field testing.

The patient whose threshold-related 120 point screen is shown in Figure 5-16 presented with a 2-day history of headache and blurred vision. The visual field was ordered because a defect on the right side was detected by confrontation testing. The screening test reveals multiple misses on the right side of the visual field, suggestive of a right homonymous hemianopia, mostly involving the inferior quadrant. The pattern of the missed spots is suggestive of a posterior pathway lesion because the pattern is congruous.

The patient underwent threshold testing 26 days later, shown in Figure 5-17. Undoubtedly there has been some improvement in the field, but because the first field was not quantified it is difficult to know how much improvement occurred. The loss pattern is highly congruous and localizes the cerebral vascular accident as posterior to the occipital cortex. The central 30-2 threshold test in this case is more informative than the screening test.

Communication Within the Visual Field Testing System

Once the decision to perform a visual field test has been made, the test has been selected, and the parameters have been decided, the necessary information must be communicated to the person who will administer the test. The essential information includes how soon it is to be done, when the patient will be seen again, what test is to be done, how the test is to be done (strategy), what type of printouts and analysis are required, the distance refraction, what to do with the pupils (dilate or not), and what stimulus to use (size and color).

The way this information is communicated will vary with the complexity of the practice setting. By maintaining the records of the practice on the premises, a solo practitioner will be able to schedule the test and include the relevant information in the medical record. The record can then be made available to the perimetrist when the patient comes in for the examination.

A multi-provider practice poses more difficulty. Communication may still be via the medical record, but the assurance of proper follow-up becomes the issue. Difficulties arise in situations where the records are

Table 5-1
Suggestions for Test Selection

Type of Patient	Test Type	Array	Strategy	Stimulus Size	Follow-up
Routine examination, no complaints	visual field testing not recommended	n/a	n/a	n/a	n/a
Complains of loss of "side vision"	screen	120 point	three zone or quantify defects	III	threshold testing
Complains of "spots" in central vision	Amsler grid	n/a	n/a	n/a	n/a
	30-2, 10-2	III	full threshold	III	overview, change analysis
Glaucoma— early to moderate	threshold	30-2, 24-2	full threshold	III	glaucoma change probability
Glaucoma—advanced	threshold probability	30-2, 24-2	full threshold	III, IV	glaucoma change
Glaucoma—end stage	threshold	30-2, 24-2	full threshold	V	stimulus V overview
		10-2		III	overview, change analysis
Neurologic: detection, asymptomatic patient	screen	120 point	quantify defects	III	threshold test
Neurologic: detection, symptomatic patient	threshold	30-2	full threshold	III	overview, change analysis
Neurologic: patient requiring serial examinations	threshold	30-2	full threshold	III	overview, change analysis
Patients with Amsler grid defects	threshold	10-2	full threshold	III	overview, change analysis
Monitoring patients at risk threshold for maculopathy (eg, drug toxicity)	threshold	10-2	full threshold	III white, red	overview, change analysis
Any patient having difficulty with threshold test	threshold	24-2	FASTPAC	III	overview, change analysis
	screen	76 point	quantify defects	III	none available, can try threshold test next time
Frail, infirm, disabled patients	screen	76 point	threshold related, three zone	III	none available

not maintained in the practice. Information contained in a medical record that has the potential for not being available at the time the test is administered is the same as having no information at all.

A proposed solution to avoiding the possibility of miscommunication is to use a visual field ordering form, such as the one shown in Figure 5-18. The form is filled out when the decision is made to order a visual field. The provider indicates which type of field is desired (Humphrey or Goldmann in this practice setting), the date of the order, when the test should be done (allowing for advance scheduling to coincide with the next visit), and when the patient is to be seen again. The option of seeing the patient on the same day of the exam before the test is done is usually to allow a refractometry recheck. To reduce the number of office

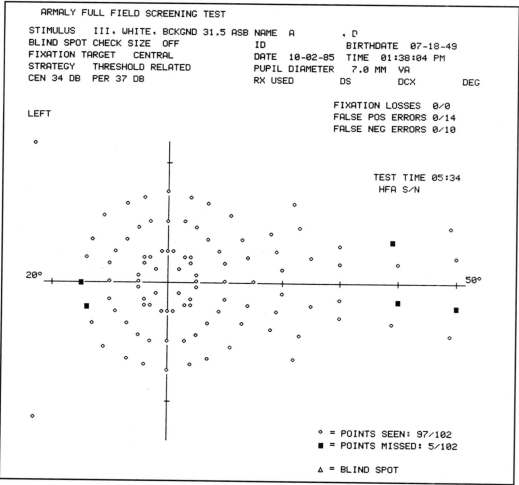

Figure 5-12. A threshold related screening test.

visits, patients requiring pupillary dilation for the visual field test are also seen before the test, allowing for pressure checks, dilation, refractometry once dilated, and fundus exam. An alternative for patients requiring dilation for the visual field is to perform a dilated examination and refractometry at the original visit and record the dilated measurement on the ordering form. Specific dilating instructions for the perimetrist should also be noted. Systems with multiple providers and locations should indicate who ordered the test and from which site.

The perimetrist must be made aware of patients who lack accommodation; therefore, the form allows for the identification of patients who are aphakic, pseudophakic, or dilated. The form also allows for the identification of patients who will be tested while wearing their own contact lenses. (Alerting the perimetrist to this prevents the use of unnecessary additional distance correction.) Once the form has been completed, it is brought to the scheduling desk for an appointment. The date and time of the appointment are noted on the top of the form, and the form is then forwarded to the visual field testing area where it is kept on file. When the patient reports for the examination, the form is pulled and all of the necessary information is then available. The bottom portion of the form allows for the technician to comment on the test performance, which is useful when interpreting the results of the test.

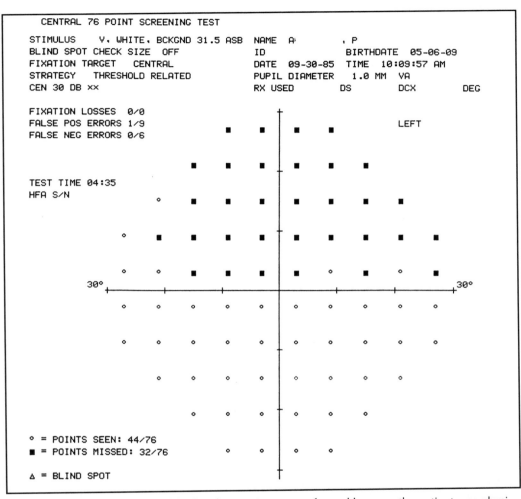

```
CENTRAL 76 POINT SCREENING TEST

STIMULUS      V, WHITE, BCKGND 31.5 ASB   NAME  A       , P
BLIND SPOT CHECK SIZE   OFF               ID                BIRTHDATE  05-06-09
FIXATION TARGET    CENTRAL                DATE  09-30-85  TIME  10:09:57 AM
STRATEGY    THRESHOLD RELATED             PUPIL DIAMETER   1.0 MM  VA
CEN 30 DB xx                              RX USED         DS        DCX         DEG

FIXATION LOSSES   0/0
FALSE POS ERRORS 1/9                                                LEFT
FALSE NEG ERRORS 0/6


TEST TIME 04:35
HFA S/N

    30°                                                             30°


° = POINTS SEEN: 44/76
■ = POINTS MISSED: 32/76

△ = BLIND SPOT
```

Figure 5-13. A 76-point threshold related screening test performed because the patient was physically incapable of performing any other type of test.

Setting up the Machine for an Examination

Step 1: Gather the Necessary Information

Automated perimeters must be set up for each examination prior to testing. The technician needs the visual field order and the patient information to proceed with the machine setup. In our system, the ordering information is found on the visual field order form, and the patient information is found on a yellow index card as previously described. If the machine is capable of using information from prior tests (either for starting subsequent tests or for performing data analysis), make sure all of the disk-based data is available and appropriately stored for use.

Step 2: Identify the Patient to the Machine

Some machines require patient information, either simply to place it on the visual field printout or in order to properly perform data analysis if such software is available. The patient's name, identification number (social security number is recommended as a unique identifier), and birth date should be entered following the manufacturer's instructions. It is important to enter the patient's name the same way every time.

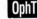

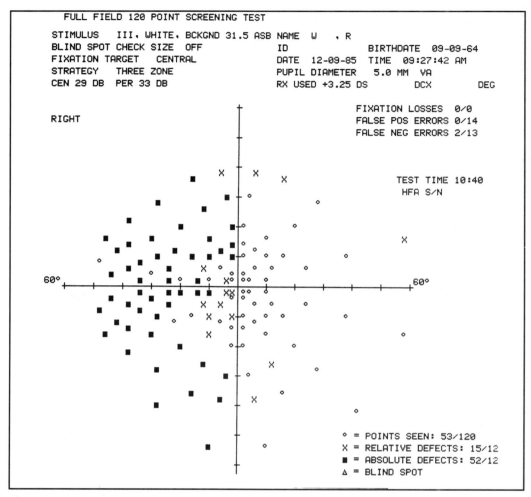

Figure 5-14. The three zone screening test.

Any alteration will cause a failure to find all of the patient's examinations for change analysis (if so equipped). Joe Smith, Joseph Smith, and Joe E. Smith are all different patients as far as the machine is concerned. Entering the correct birth date is essential for proper calculation of the add (if an automatic trial lens calculation feature is available) and to tell any analytical software how old the patient is for comparison to the correct age-matched normal population. An example of an error due to incorrect birth date entry is given in Chapter 7.

Step 3: Select the Correcting Lens

Because a visual field test requires the patient to discern an often faint test object against a lighted background, the chances of the patient seeing the stimulus are increased if the stimulus is in focus. You must know the size of the perimeter bowl in order to properly focus the image of the stimulus (consult the user's manual). Unless the perimeter operates at "optical infinity" like the Octopus 1-2-3®, an addition will be required. The power of the add, and thus the power of the correcting lens, is based on the patient's distance refractometric measurement. The technician should not rely on reading the glasses the patient is wearing to determine the correcting lens, however, because patients may show up for the test without them, or the pre-

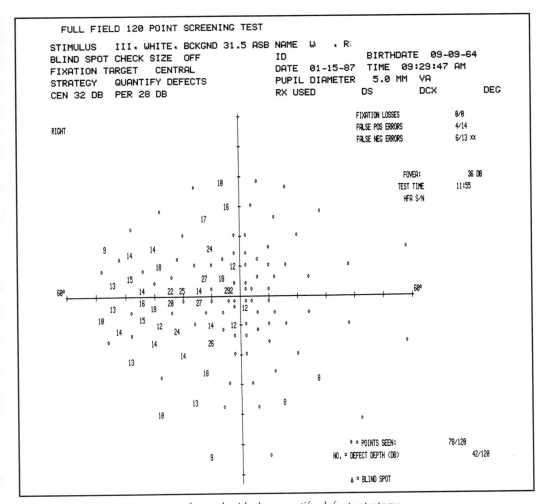

Figure 5-15. A screening test performed with the quantify defects strategy.

scription may have been changed and the new glasses have not yet been picked up. Distance refractometry should be recent and appropriate to the test situation. Ideally, the visual acuity should be checked with this measurement to assure that the acuity is at its known best. If not, and the acuity improves with a pinhole, you will need to perform refractometry prior to the visual field. All patients undergoing dilation for the visual field test must have post-dilation, refractometry, either just prior to the visual field test or at a recent previous visit. (Patients with pupils less than 2 mm should be dilated for the visual field test. The full near add of +3.00 diopters is then used over the dilated measurement.) Once the distance refractometric measurement is established, the lens to be used must be calculated.

The simplest method for lens selection is to use the machine's automatic lens calculation feature, if available in the operating software. If the software does not allow automatic calculation, the lens must be calculated manually based on the distance prescription and the patient's age. Table 5-2 summarizes the steps used for selecting the trial lens, assuming a bowl size of 33 cm.

The small inset table showing the age-specific adds should be copied and taped to the side of the field analyzer or to the trial lens set for ready reference. Remember to use the add as specified by the manufacturer, not the add found in the patient's glasses. Often patients read at distances greater than 1/3 m and thus will not be corrected for the distance of the visual field test. Don't forget to perform the trial lens calculations for each

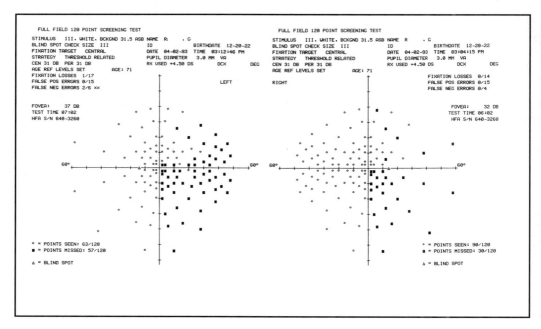

Figure 5-16. An incongruous right homonymous hemianopic defect detected on a 120-point screening test performed with the threshold related strategy.

eye separately. Table 5-3 gives a few examples of trial lens calculations for the Humphrey Field Analyzer.

Once the correcting lens has been determined, insert the lens(es) into the lens holder, with the sphere in the slot closest to the patient and the cylinder, oriented to the correct axis, in the far slot. Make sure the lenses used are the rimless variety, as ordinary trial lenses have thick rims which will block out a portion of the patient's visual field, leading to artificial loss. The correcting lens and holder must be removed when testing any portion of the visual field outside of the central 30°. If a test pattern includes points both within and outside of the central 30°, the machine will pause when testing of the central 30° is completed and prompt the technician to remove the lens prior to proceeding with the peripheral field.

The effect of incorrect lenses will be discussed further in Chapter 7. Patients should be encouraged to advise the technician if the interior of the machine seems out of focus.

One good indication that the lens was incorrect may be gleaned from a measurement of the foveal threshold. This option may be selected for threshold tests performed with the Humphrey Field Analyzer. The patient is instructed to fixate within the center of an illuminated diamond below the usual fixation spot. The foveal threshold is then determined by projecting stimuli into the center of the diamond. An abnormally low foveal threshold in a patient known to have good visual acuity and no macular pathology almost always indicates that the patient was not properly focused within the bowl.

Step 4: Select the Test

The visual field ordering sheet or the medical record should contain all of the test parameters desired by the clinician. Select the appropriate options according to the operating instructions for your machine. Make sure the machine is configured to perform the test as ordered. The machine should now be ready for the patient. Remember that frequently used configurations and setups can be added to user-defined menus if available so that it will not be necessary to go through all of the above steps to set up the machine each time a patient is tested.

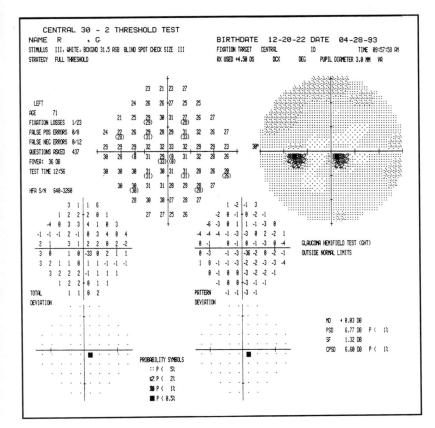

Figure 5-17. The 30-2 threshold test of the same patient as in Figure 5-16, 26 days later.

Patient Set-up

Patient Instructions

While the machine is being set up, the patient should have the opportunity to become familiar with the test procedures. A printed information sheet is most helpful for preparing the patient. Patients tend to be anxious while undergoing medical examinations, and this may be true especially when the test is unfamiliar and foreign. The patient may have been told that he or she has been scheduled for a test and not have any idea what it is about. Maximizing the patient's understanding of the procedure (what it is for, how it is performed, what he or she is supposed to do, and what to expect during the test) can help reduce apprehension. It is especially important to tell the patient in advance that there will be periods of time during the test when the lights will be too dim to be seen as the machine attempts to determine how sensitive the eyes are. This helps reduce the patient's feeling that he or she must be blind because the light can't be seen. Another important point to emphasize is that the patient has the ability to rest when needed by holding down the response button. This will alert the technician that a rest period is desired and the test can be paused.

date scheduled: _____
time scheduled: _____

Visual Field Order Form

[] Humphrey [] Goldmann   phone:

ADDRESSOGRAPH STAMP

Instructions for using this form: All **required** information indicated in bold. No test
will be scheduled if this information is not supplied. Indicate choices by circling when choices are listed or by placing check marks in appropriate
spaces.

date exam ordered: _____
date exam desired: __ routine in ___ month(s) / week(s)   __add-on ASAP
                  __ today (emergency)   __other (specify exact date) _____
next appointment with provider:
    __ same day as field (before / after)
    __ anytime after field within _____ week(s) / month(s)

provider: _____   location: NMCSD ophth / NMCSD optom / region

Test desired: Threshold: 30-2 / 24-2 / 10-2   Strategy: full threshold / full from prior
    __ other threshold test (specify) _____
    __ 120 point screen Strategy: threshold related / three-zone / quantify defects
    __ other screening test (and strategy) _____
    __ Goldmann: screening / glaucoma / neurological

Printout for threshold tests (if other than standard STATPAC single field analysis):
    __ value table / graytone / defect depth / triple (includes all three formats)
    __ profile (specify cut) _____
    __ compare with last visual field
    __ glaucoma change probability   Prior visual field here? [] yes [] no

    distance refraction: OD   _____-_____x_____ aphakic / dilated / contacts
                        OS   _____-_____x_____ aphakic / dilated / contacts

    __ non-standard stimulus size (default = III): ___ OD ___ OS
    __ non-standard stimulus color (default = white): red / blue / green
    __ patient to be dilated for exam using:
          __ 1% Mydriacyl x __ __ OD __ OS   V$_A$ OD _____ A$_T$ OD ____
          __ 2.5% Neo. x ___ __ OD __ OS   OS   OS
(Technician note: dilated or aphakic patients require full add. All others, including contact lens patients, require appropriate add for age as specified
in the manual. Record visual acuity and intraocular pressure prior to instilling dilating drops.)

Technician comments: Patient understood test?   yes / no
                   Required constant supervision?   yes / no
                   Exhibited good fixation behavior?   yes / no
                   Complained?   yes / no
                   Rested frequently?   yes / no
                   Required larger stimulus than ordered?   yes / no

    Other comments/observations: _____

                   (At completion of exam, attach this form to printout) tech initial: _____

Figure 5-18. Example of a visual field ordering form.

Table 5-2
Determining the Correcting Lens

1. Ignore cylinder powers of less than 0.25 diopters. Calculate spherical equivalent power for lenses with cylinder between 0.25 and 1.50 diopters (to calculate spherical equivalent power, add half the cylinder power to that of the sphere, then ignore the cylinder). Use the full cylinder for cylinders greater than 1.50 diopters. This determines the resultant lens.

2. Determine the add required based on age or accommodation from the chart:

Patient's Age	Add Needed
<30	no add
30-39	+1.00
40-44	+1.50
45-49	+2.00
50-54	+2.50
>55	+3.00
aphakic, pseudophakic, or dilated (any age): +3.00	

3. Add the resultant distance lens to the age-required add. This is the lens to be used.

Table 5-3
Examples of Trial Lens Calculations

Patient's Age	Distance Rfx	Cylinder Action	Resultant Rfx	Accommodative State	Add Based on Age or Accommodation	Lens Used for Test
29	-1.75-0.25 X 175	ignore	-1.75 sph	normal	+0.00	-1.75 sph
32	-1.75-1.00 X 145	add ½ to sph	-2.25 sph	normal	+1.00	-1.25 sph
54	+2.25-2.00 X 90	use full	+2.25-2.00 X 90	normal	+2.50	+4.75-2.00 X 90
52,	-1.00-3.00 X 105 on pilo	use full	-1.00-3.00 X 105	dilated for exam = none	+3.00	+2.00-3.00 X 105
72	+4.00-1.00 X 85	add ½ to sph	+3.50 sph	normal	+3.00	+6.50 sph
53	+2.00-4.00 X 70 pseudophake	use full	+2.00-4.00 X 70	none -	+3.00	+5.00-4.00 X 70

Rx = prescription; sph = spherical; pilo =pilocarpine.

What the Patient Needs to Know

- This is a test of your side or peripheral vision.

- We test one eye at a time, so one eye will be covered.

- When I start the test, your chin will be in the cup and your forehead against this bar. Your job for the entire test is to look at this light here in the middle. As you look in the center, another light will come on somewhere inside the bowl. When you first think you see this "extra" light, press this button.

- You won't see the target light all the time. Sometimes you may seem to go for a long time without seeing anything. Don't worry; just be patient until the light appears again. The main thing is not to look for the light. Always look right here in the center.

- Don't wait trying to be sure whether you see the light or not. Press the button when you first think you see it. Any areas that seem inconsistent will be rechecked.

- I have a little screen that shows me your eye. If I notice that you are looking around instead of at the center, I'll remind you to look straight ahead. If the machine catches you looking around, it will beep.

- From time to time you'll feel your head move slightly as I keep your position adjusted.

- If you need to rest, hold down the response button.

- Be sure not to stare. You can blink whenever you need to.

- If you are uncomfortable, let me know.

Other points to emphasize include information that needs to be communicated to the operator so that adjustments in the test situation can be made. If the patients don't tell the technician that they are uncomfortable or that the inside of the bowl is not in focus, the test will proceed and obtain meaningless results. Such patients will certainly not be happy hearing that the test needs to be repeated.

All instructions should be reinforced verbally and repeated as often as necessary both before and during the test to make sure that the patient understands and is performing as well as possible. Patients with prior automated fields should still read the instructions prior to each test in order to reinforce the above information. There is a learning effect in automated perimetry, and it may take up to four examinations before a patient is fully "seasoned." Written and verbal instructions, repeated as necessary as the test proceeds, may help to flatten the learning curve for the patient and make the results more accurate and reliable. On-screen instructions are also available. Reading such instructions to each patient at every test serves to standardize the procedures, even with different examiners. Table 5-4 is a sample visual field instruction sheet for patients. Feel free to copy it as is or adapt it for your practice.

Positioning

Once the machine and the patient are ready, the patient must be properly positioned. The patient should be seated comfortably on a reasonably soft chair with the neck, shoulders, and arms relaxed. The machine should be at such a height that the patient's forehead is in contact with the headrest when the chin is placed into the chinrest, with no tendency to fall back. Figure 5-19 shows a patient improperly positioned in the machine. The positioning in Figure 5-20 also is incorrect, as the table is too low. This patient will become uncomfortable in a short time due to the forced hunching of the shoulders and kinking of the neck. Figure 5-21, although at first glance appearing to be all right, shows the effect of the table being too

---

Table 5-4
Visual Field Instructions

Your doctor has ordered a visual field examination for you. This test determines the sensitivity of your peripheral vision, that is, how well you see "out of the corner of your eye". The examination will be performed by a computerized machine known as the Humphrey Field Analyzer, which is among the most advanced methods available today for measuring the visual field. The examination is not difficult, but there are some aspects of it with which you should be familiar. Please read this material prior to your examination.

Because this is an examination of your "side" vision, it is most important that you hold your eye still and look straight ahead at all times. Inside the machine there is a steady yellow light for you to look at. Unless instructed otherwise, you should stare at this light at all times. The test lights will flash on and off randomly at different places within the machine. You will be given a response button to hold, and you should press the button whenever you think you have seen a light flash. The best time to blink is right after you have pushed the button. Some lights will be bright and some will be dim; some lights will be too dim to be seen and there will be periods of time when you won't see anything. Don't be alarmed by this—the machine purposely makes some of the lights too dim as it tries to measure the sensitivity of your eye at various points.

During the examination, you will hear various noises as the light projector moves and the shutter opens and closes. Try to ignore these noises and respond only to the lights—the machine periodically tests your responses either by not projecting any lights (to see if you are responding to the noises) or by projecting very bright lights (to see if you are paying attention).

This examination can be quite long and tiring, and can take up to 20 minutes per eye. It is most important that you be seated comfortably with your forehead pushed forward into the machine as far as possible. You should feel relaxed with no tension in your shoulders or neck. The fixation light should be clearly in focus. If you are not comfortable or if the light is not in focus, tell the technician immediately. If you wish to rest during the examination simply hold down the response button—the machine will beep and alert the technician to pause the test.

It is hoped that this information will make visual field testing easier for you. Please do not hesitate to ask the technician or your doctor to explain anything that is not clear to you.

---

high. The patient has to stretch her neck to reach the head strap. Shortly after beginning the test her head will fall away from the machine, leaving a large space between her eye and the correcting lens. This can lead to artifactual visual field loss. The patient shown in Figure 5-22 is positioned properly, with the machine set at the proper height.

Once the table height is set and the patient is seated properly, have the patient sit back. Place the occluder over the non-tested eye, making sure that the eye is completely covered and that the elastic strap does not cover the eye being tested. Reposition the patient in the machine and adjust the chinrest height and position so that the tested eye is properly centered as indicated by the monitoring system of your machine. The correcting lens is then brought as close as possible to the eye without touching it or the eyelashes. Figure 5-23 shows what can happen if the correcting lens is not properly positioned. The lens holder in this case was too high (or the eye too low), allowing the black casing of the lens holder to block out the inferior portion of the visual field. This may be mistaken for loss due to disease. Other examples of lens malpositioning and correcting lens artifact are given in Chapter 7.

Once everything seems ready, ask the patient if he or she feels comfortable and if the fixation target is in focus. Make any necessary corrections prior to proceeding. Make sure the patient understands what is going to happen and run the demonstration program if necessary. When the patient voices an understanding of the procedure, begin the test. Figure 5-24 shows the appearance of the monitoring screen and the video eye monitor of a Humphrey Field Analyzer with a patient and the correcting lens properly positioned, ready for the test to begin.

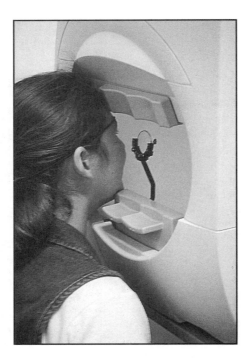

Figure 5-19. Patient improperly positioned in the Humphrey Field Analyzer.

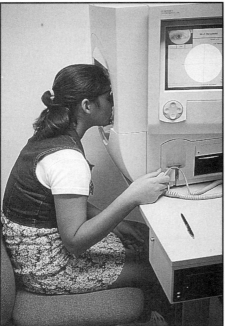

Figure 5-20. Table too low, forcing the patient to bend too far.

Administering the Test

OptA

OptT

OphT

The patient must never be left alone during the actual examination. Performance should be monitored by whatever means are available on your machine. Watch closely for false positive and negative errors, and reinstruct the patient after each error. For example, if the patient has just made a false positive error (indicating that he or she pushed the response button when no stimulus had been projected), remind him or her

Figure 5-21. Table too high, forcing the patient to stretch her neck. Note how the forehead has drifted back from the headrest.

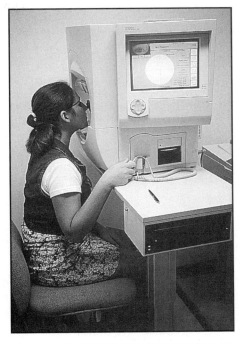

Figure 5-22. Table height set just right for the patient.

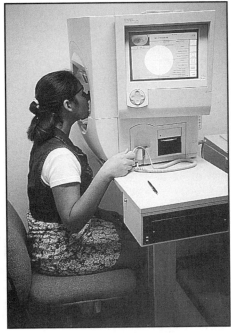

to push the button only when a light is seen. Similarly, if a false negative error is made (indicating that the patient failed to push the button when a bright stimulus was flashed in an area that the machine has already determined to have vision), check to make sure that the patient is paying attention, is comfortable, does not want to rest, etc. Periodic coaching and encouragement, such as "You're doing fine, Mrs. Jones," or "Just a few more minutes to go," can be extremely helpful in increasing the patient's level of comfort.

The technician must be more than a baby sitter during the performance of the test. Even though the

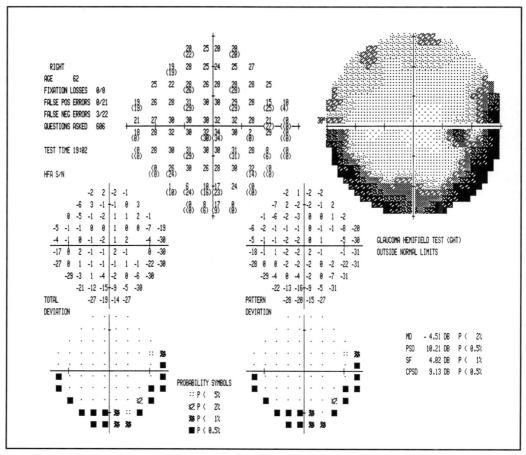

Figure 5-23. The lens holder artifact, resulting from positioning the correcting lens too high relative to the patient's eye.

machine may use a sophisticated algorithm to monitor fixation, it is important for the operator to carefully monitor the patient's fixation as well. The patient's eye should remain centered at all times. It is natural for the patient to look toward the projected stimulus, but this should occur *after* the response button was pushed and be followed by a rapid shift back to the fixation target. If a lot of random eye movements are observed, remind the patient to try to look steadily at the fixation target. If, despite what appears to be rock-steady fixation, a machine capable of monitoring fixation continues to record fixation losses, the blind spot may be incorrectly located or it may be that the blind spot check size is too large. The technician should pause the test and remap the blind spot, and if the fixation losses persist, change the blind spot check size to a smaller stimulus, such as a I or II. Performing fixation loss catch trials with a stimulus size I does not affect the performance of the visual field test with a size III. This is discussed in more detail in Chapter 7.

Finally, a test should not be allowed to proceed if the patient does not appear to be responding to the stimuli. If the patient understands the test procedure and has advanced visual field loss, a field full of zeros is worthless. The test should be stopped and restarted with a larger stimulus, such as size V. Similarly, a patient who proves to be physically incapable of performing a full threshold test should be tried with a simpler test, such as a screen. The decision to deviate from the requested test is that of the operator and is based on the patient's ability. If in doubt, check with the ordering provider prior to continuing. Any changes from the ordered examination should be fully documented and explained in the medical record then signed and dated by the examiner.

Figure 5-24. Patient and correcting lens properly positioned for the start of the test.

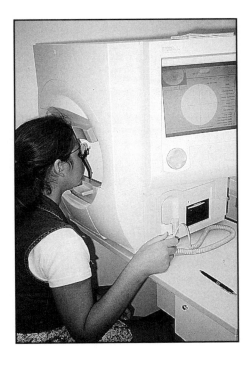

After the Test

Immediately after the test has concluded, save the results if the machine uses storage media and storage is not automatic. Data saved but later determined to be unnecessary can be deleted, but data not saved can never be recovered.

After allowing the patient to rest for as long as necessary, proceed with testing the other eye. Again, don't forget to ensure centration (and accuracy) of the correcting lens and proper positioning of the patient. Save the results at the conclusion of the test, and print out the results according to clinician request. Most machines have built in printers, while others may require the data to be downloaded to an external computer for processing, formatting, and printing. Some machines allow "batch" printing of multiple examinations so that if the results of a test are not required immediately, many tests may be printed over a lunch hour or overnight. Consult the owner's manual of your machine for specific instructions on how to print.

Table 5-5 lists the various printout options for central threshold tests for the Humphrey Field Analyzer. All patients should have some sort of single field printout. Most patients, particularly glaucoma patients and those under treatment for neurological disease, should have some sort of change over time printout. The type of printout(s) desired should be specified by the clinician when the test is ordered.

Finally, the technician should record comments on the visual field order form or document the performance in the medical record. Items of particular importance are fixation behavior, understanding of the test, cooperation, attitude, and anything else that is felt to be important. The order form with the comments and technician's initials should be placed in the patient's chart along with the field printouts for review by the provider. Notes written in the record by the technician should be signed and dated.

A Checklist for Visual Field Technicians

1. Pull the patient's yellow card from the file or create a new one if the patient is new. Fill in all information.
2. Check the visual field order form for appropriate information, including refractometric measured to be used.

OptA

OptT

OphT

OptA

OptT

OphT

Table 5-5
Printout Options for the Humphrey Field Analyzer

Printout Type	Features	Example Figure No.
Single Field Printouts		
Value Table	Numeric grid of threshold values	5-25
Defect Depth (non-STATPAC)	Algebraic difference between measured threshold values and the *expected* normal values	5-26
Graytone	Graphic representation of the threshold values generated by assigning symbols of increasing darkness corresponding to decreasing sensitivity	5-27
Three-in-One (non-STATPAC)	Includes value table, defect depth, and graytone	5-28
Profile (non-STATPAC)	Static cut through a meridian specified by the operator	5-29
STATPAC (software option, two versions)	Includes standard value table and graytone, adds total deviation plot (algebraic difference between measured threshold values and an *age-corrected normal* database), pattern deviation plot (highlighting focal loss over diffuse loss), probability plots for observed deviations, visual field indices (mean deviation, pattern standard deviation, short-term fluctuation, corrected pattern standard deviation), and (in version B) the glaucoma hemifield test (designed to detect asymmetric loss across the horizontal midline)	5-30
Change Over Time Printouts (STATPAC software only)		
Overview	Graytone, value table, total deviation probability plot, and pattern deviation probability plot displayed for up to 16 tests on a single printout printed in chronological order from earliest to most recent examination	5-31
Change Analysis	Graphical representation of reduced data for all tests performed, includes "box plot" (a histogram of the total deviation plot) and plots of each of the four indices	5-32
Glaucoma Probability Plot (STATPAC II only)	Takes first two examinations as baseline and compares each subsequent examination to the baseline, showing numeric change of each point from baseline and compares the observed changes to a population of "clinically stable" glaucoma patients	5-33

3. Set up the machine for the test using information on the patient data card and the order form. Place the corrective lens in the holder, using age appropriate add on top of specified distance measurement. If dilated or aphakic use +3.00 add.

4. Position the patient. Make sure the table height and chinrest are adjusted properly to assure patient comfort. Ask if the patient is comfortable and make appropriate corrections.

5. Measure pupil size and record on the patient data screen.

6. Enter patient information into the machine, including optic data and pupil size. Make sure birth date and year are correct (do not enter test year). Make sure patient's name is entered identically to previous tests.

7. Patient should have read the handout "Visual Field Testing—Information for Patients." Instruct the patient as to the nature of test and its performance. Read the instructions to the patient from

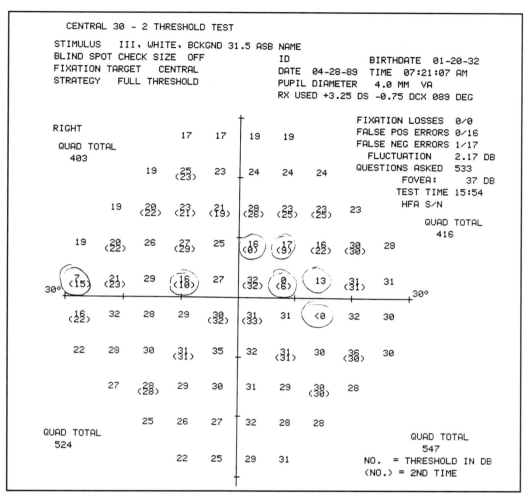

```
CENTRAL 30 - 2 THRESHOLD TEST

STIMULUS    III. WHITE. BCKGND 31.5 ASB NAME
BLIND SPOT CHECK SIZE   OFF          ID                 BIRTHDATE  01-20-32
FIXATION TARGET    CENTRAL           DATE   04-28-89  TIME   07:21:07 AM
STRATEGY    FULL THRESHOLD           PUPIL DIAMETER    4.0 MM   VA
                                     RX USED +3.25 DS -0.75 DCX 089 DEG
```

Figure 5-25. The value table printout.

the machine. Make sure the patient understands the procedure and answer any questions before proceeding.

8. Make sure the patient understands the anticipated length of the test and knows how to rest by holding down the response button.

9. Occlude the untested eye, reposition the patient, check the position of the corrective lens, recheck the patient's position, make the necessary adjustments, and proceed.

10. Every 1 or 2 minutes check the patient's fixation and position. Pause and make adjustments as necessary.

11. **Never leave the room for any reason while a test is being performed. Monitor the patient and the screen at all times.**

12. Reinstruct the patient every time a false positive or false negative response occurs, or if fixation deviation is noted. Offer periodic encouragement and reassurance. Advise when close to finish.

13. **Save the results.**

14. Allow brief rest period and proceed with the other eye. Go back to Step 3.

15. At the conclusion of the second eye, print the results according to the order form. Answer the questions at the bottom of the order form and make any comments deemed necessary. Place the printouts and the order form in the patient's chart.

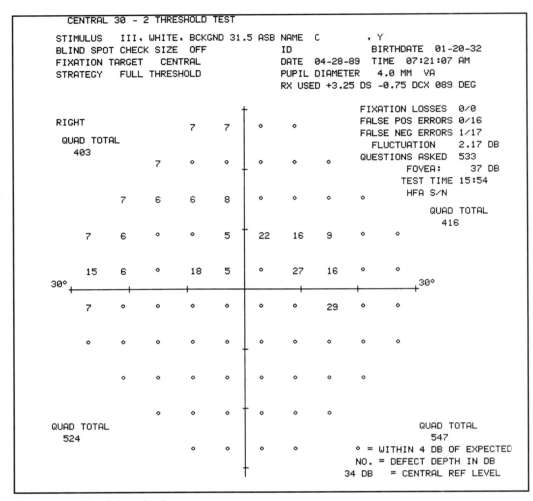

Figure 5-26. The defect depth printout.

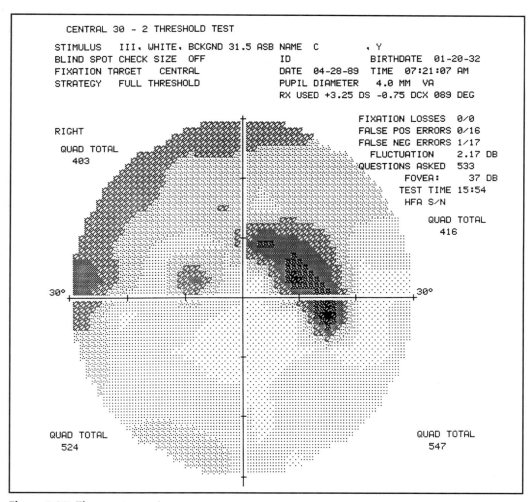

Figure 5-27. The graytone printout.

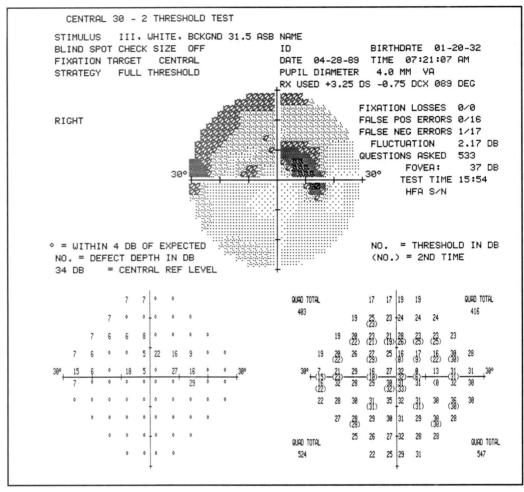

Figure 5-28. The "three-in-one" printout.

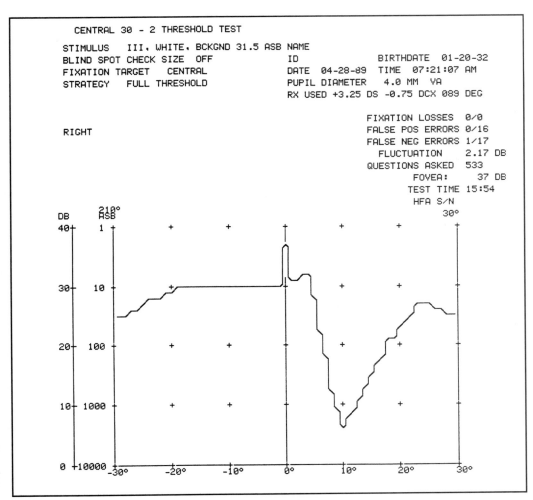

```
CENTRAL 30 - 2 THRESHOLD TEST

STIMULUS    III, WHITE, BCKGND 31.5 ASB NAME
BLIND SPOT CHECK SIZE   OFF          ID                   BIRTHDATE   01-20-32
FIXATION TARGET    CENTRAL           DATE  04-28-89  TIME  07:21:07 AM
STRATEGY    FULL THRESHOLD           PUPIL DIAMETER   4.0 MM   VA
                                     RX USED +3.25 DS -0.75 DCX 089 DEG

                                          FIXATION LOSSES   0/0
         RIGHT                            FALSE POS ERRORS  0/16
                                          FALSE NEG ERRORS  1/17
                                             FLUCTUATION      2.17 DB
                                          QUESTIONS ASKED   533
                                                 FOVEA:         37 DB
                                             TEST TIME 15:54
                                                HFA S/N
        210°                                                   30°
DB      ASB
40+     1 +    +      +      +     +      +      +     +
```

Figure 5-29. A static cut giving a profile of the island of vision.

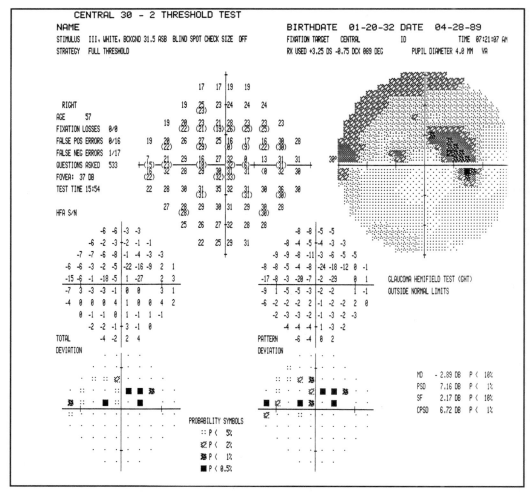

Figure 5-30. The STATPAC single field analysis.

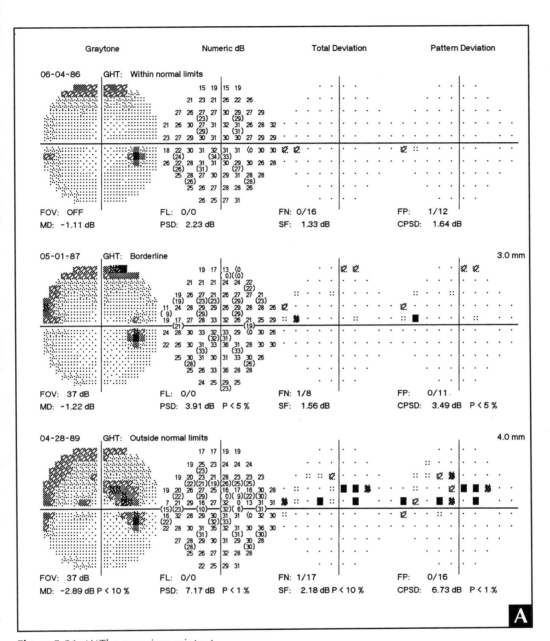

Figure 5-31. (A)The overview printout.

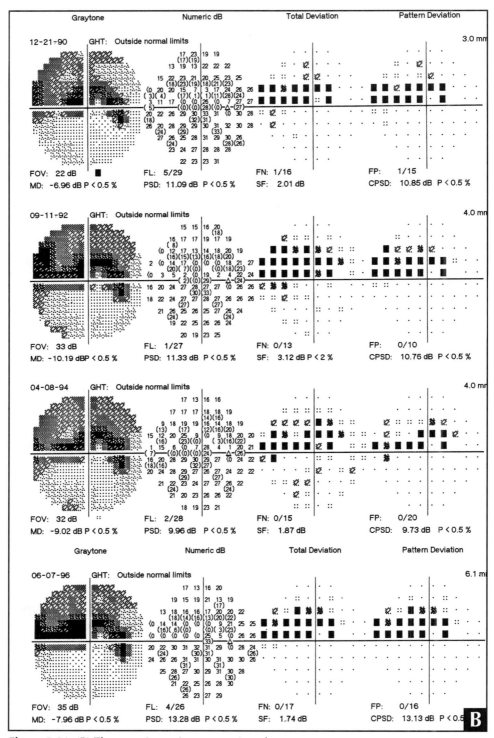

Figure 5-31. (B) The overview printout, continued.

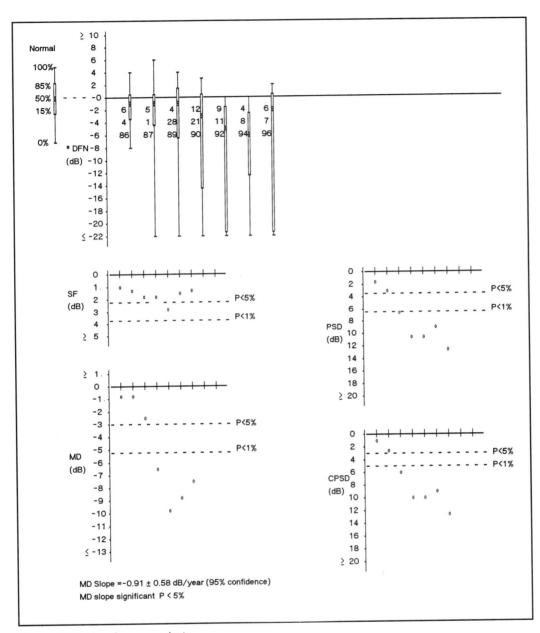

Figure 5-32. The change analysis.

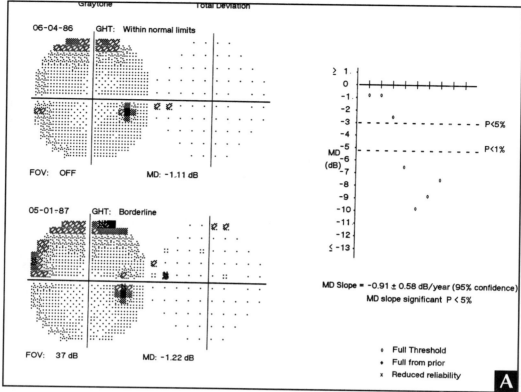

Figure 5-33. The glaucoma change probability plot.

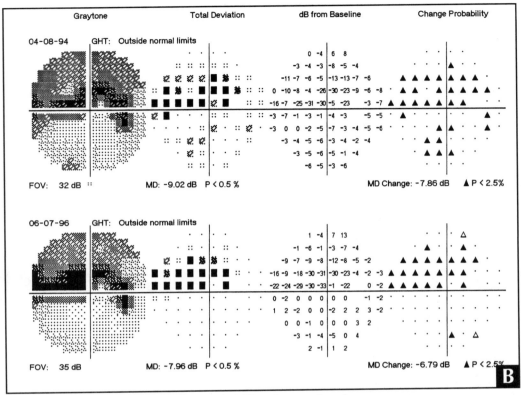

Figure 5-33. (B)The glaucoma change probablility plot, continued.

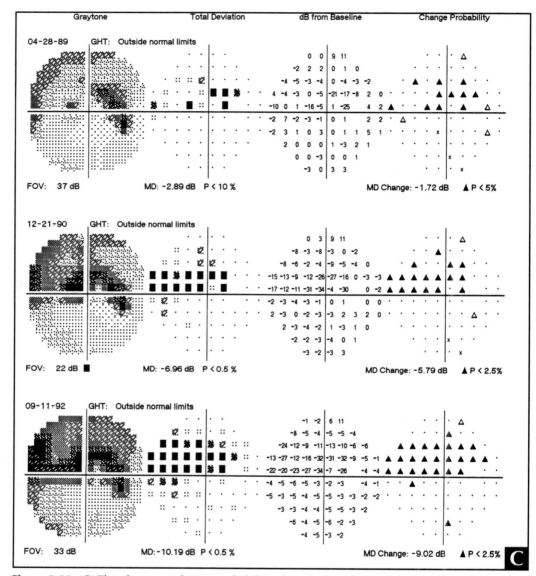

Figure 5-33. (C) The glaucoma change probability plot, continued.

Chapter 6

Special Test Techniques

KEY POINTS

- Shallow central or paracentral scotomas that might otherwise be missed can frequently be detected and characterized using color test objects.

- Reliable results can be obtained from visual field testing of patients with poor central vision when adequate fixation targets are provided.

- Common findings in non-physiologic visual loss include spiral visual fields on Goldmann perimetry and "tunnel" or non-expanding fields when tested at varying distances on the tangent screen.

- Binocular field testing is used to evaluate the extent of diplopia.

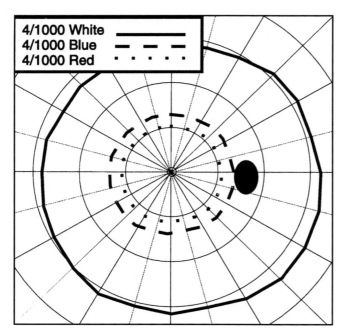

4/1000 White ———
4/1000 Blue — — —
4/1000 Red • • • • •

Figure 6-1. Normal tangent screen findings when testing with white, red, and blue test objects.

Introduction

The usual methods of visual field testing have been discussed in the preceding chapters. This chapter will deal with a variety of less commonly encountered circumstances associated with visual field testing. The use of colored test objects, visual field characteristics of non-physiologic visual loss, and measuring double vision with perimetry will be discussed, as well as testing patients who are difficult to position, those with poor vision, and those with ptosis. These situations present challenges to the perimetrist above and beyond those encountered in more routine visual field testing.

Colored Targets

Most often the visual field is explored using white test objects. There are occasions, however, in which testing with color is useful.

There are several factors that allow color visual field testing to provide information not easily obtained with the more conventional white test objects. Colored test objects reflect less light than white test objects of the same size; mapping the field with colored tangent screen objects is therefore similar to testing with white test objects of similar size under varying illumination conditions. In addition, the sensitivity of the retina varies with the color of the stimulus, assuming equal luminance, and in some disease states the relative sensitivities are altered.

Many methods for testing the visual field can make use of color. Amsler testing with the red grid was discussed in Chapter 3. Red bottle caps from mydriatic drops can be used in confrontation testing to screen for shallow central scotomas.

Tangent screen perimetry can be performed using any color of test target, as can the Autoplot™. When performing color tangent screen perimetry, red test objects are most commonly used. Other frequently used colors are blue and green. In performing the test with colored objects, it is best to plot isopters with targets that vary in color, but are the same size. Typically, the isopter determined with a colored test object is smaller than that obtained with a similarly-sized white object, and the isopter plotted with red is smaller than the one obtained with blue (Figure 6-1). The methods used for tangent screen testing with colored test objects are the same as those described for white test objects in the section on tangent screen testing in Chapter 3.

The Humphrey Field Analyzer has filters for testing with red, green, blue, and yellow. Short wavelength automated perimetry (SWAP), found on some newer models of the Humphrey Field Analyzer, uses blue stimuli projected on a yellow background and may detect glaucomatous changes in the visual field earlier than standard automated perimetry. (SWAP will be discussed in more detail in Chapter 11.) The Goldmann perimeter can be configured with color filters for color perimetry as well.

Abnormalities in a variety of disorders can be determined using color visual field evaluation. Shallow central scotomas in mild optic neuropathy or early macular disease may be more easily measured using red test objects than with the standard white. A simple screening method is to hold a red bottle cap in front of the patient and alternately cover the patient's eyes, asking if the color is equally "good." If an optic neuropathy is present, the color on the abnormal side will often be described as faded, washed out, pale, dimmer, or darker than the other side. Blue may be useful in central serous retinopathy. In dominant optic atrophy of Kjerr (an inherited disorder), the isopter to blue is smaller than the isopter to red, a reversal of the normal finding. Many practitioners test for toxicity of the drug hydroxychloroquine (Plaquenil™) using a red test stimulus in a central 10° static threshold test on an automated perimeter.

Physical Disabilities

It may be difficult to use standard visual field testing techniques in bedridden patients or those with physical disabilities or deformities. Sometimes it will be impossible to position the patient in order to obtain reliable bowl perimetry. Patients with restrictive strabismus, as is commonly found in Graves' dysthyroid ophthalmopathy, may not be able to maintain fixation on the central fixation target when positioned in bowl perimeters. A similar problem arises in patients with neck problems such as torticollis or cervical spine arthritis. At other times, the patient may not be able to concentrate long enough to participate in a detailed mapping of the visual field. In these situations, alternate methods will be required to obtain visual field information that is useful.

Wheelchair

Some automated perimeters have been designed to facilitate testing of patients in wheelchairs (Figure 6-2). If a wheelchair-bound patient cannot be properly positioned for bowl perimetry, careful tangent screen testing usually can be performed. In either situation, it is important to position the patient so that the fixation target can be viewed comfortably.

Bedridden Patients

Bedridden patients provide an additional challenge. Usually confrontational fields must suffice. With some preparation, however, tangent screen perimetry can also be done. To accomplish this, prepare a 4 ft square black felt cloth. This cloth can be rolled or folded and taken to the bedside. The cloth can be fastened to the ceiling or hung in front of the patient if he or she can sit up in bed. Target presentation is done in the usual manner. Remember, the lighting in this situation cannot be standardized so fields obtained in this manner cannot be closely followed over time, although large changes in field defects can be trusted.

Low Vision Patients

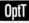

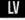

Patients with poor vision or severe visual loss present a challenge to the perimetrist. These patients may present with a variety of visual field abnormalities, based on the underlying cause of the visual loss. Of all the patterns of field loss that may be encountered, the central scotoma is the most troublesome as it wreaks

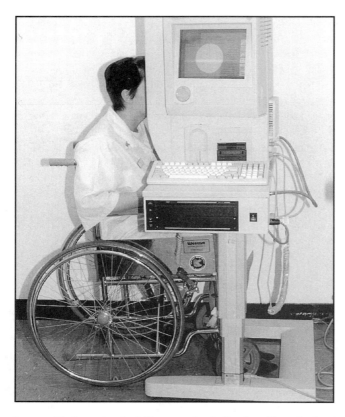

Figure 6-2. Bowl perimeter with wheelchair access.

havoc with the patient's ability to maintain fixation. If steady fixation can be achieved, reliable information can be obtained in visual field testing.

Techniques to ensure steady fixation vary with the testing method. For Amsler grid testing, the grid with the white diagonal lines is used and the patient is instructed to fixate where the lines intersect. This technique has been carried over to tangent screen visual field testing by fashioning a large "X" or cross out of white tape and attaching it to the fixation button on the tangent screen (Figure 6-3). The Humphrey Field Analyzer has four fixation lights arranged in a diamond pattern that can be used for patients with central scotomas instead of the standard central fixation light. In all these cases, the main idea is to present a visual target which the patient can use to direct and maintain fixation in a location that is obscured by a scotoma.

Non-physiologic Field Loss

Non-physiologic visual loss (also called non-organic or functional visual loss) is defined as loss of visual function where there is no lesion or organic basis to explain it. Patients exhibiting this type of visual dysfunction may have a psychiatric illness such as hysteria. But more often the patient perceives some secondary gain, as may be seen in the victim of a minor head injury who feigns loss of vision to try to win a personal injury lawsuit or to acquire workman's compensation. In children it is often a behavior expressed when there is significant stress in their lives, for example impending divorce or social/academic difficulties at school.

The tangent screen is a handy tool to establish non-physiologic field loss. The most commonly used method is to plot an isopter at 1 m and then retest at 2 m using a target twice the size of the one used at 1 m. Because the more distant test object projects the same size image on the retina as the smaller, closer target, the fields should measure the same in degrees. Note that the isopter will appear larger on the more distant screen because each degree of eccentricity is displaced twice as far on the 2 m screen as on the 1 m

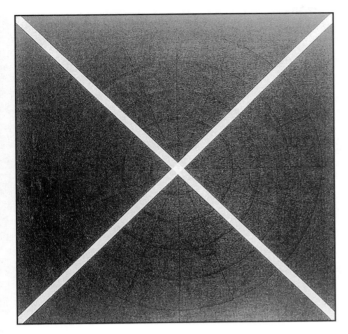

Figure 6-3. White tape "X" on a tangent screen used to improve fixation in low vision patients with central scotomas.

screen (Figure 6-4). The isopter plotted at 2 m extends exactly twice the distance from the center as the isopter plotted with a target half its size at 1 m; both isopters subtend the same visual angle.

In non-physiologic visual field loss the isopter plotted at 2 m will frequently lie at the same distance from fixation (that is, at half the visual angle) as the isopter plotted at 1 m. It is not unusual to find the 2 m isopter lying within the 1 m plot if the disorder is bona fide. Distances other than 1 m and 2 m may be used, but it is important to ensure that the test objects subtend the same visual angle regardless of the test distance.

Figure 6-5 demonstrates a non-expanding or "tunnel field." Note that the isopter plotted at 2 m is the same distance from the center of the screen and subtends a smaller visual angle than the isopter plotted at 1 m. If the patient has good acuity and the test object is very large, maintaining a constant visual angle in the target may not be critical. An example of this situation can be seen when using confrontation testing by bringing the examiner's hand in from the side and the patient does not see it until it gets to the examiner's face. If this happens when testing up close *and* from across the room, the patient is demonstrating a non-expanding field.

Spiral visual fields are another example of non-physiologic visual field abnormality. Repeat testing of a region with the same test object should yield a result that lies at about the same eccentricity as the first presentation. Patients with non-organic abnormalities will frequently respond with ever-decreasing eccentricities on repeat testing using the same stimulus. When the responses are plotted, it yields a field with a spiraling "isopter" (Figure 6-6). The spiral appearance is characteristic for non-physiologic visual field loss.

If a patient suspected of having non-physiologic visual loss has a distinctive visual field abnormality in one eye and not the other, the test may be repeated binocularly. Under physiologic circumstances, the scotoma, hemianopia, or altitudinal abnormality should disappear on binocular testing because the eye with the normal field will see the stimulus. In non-physiologic visual loss, the scotoma frequently persists and sometimes even appears to worsen under binocular conditions.

Ptosis

Patients with ptosis of the upper eyelid or the eyebrow may complain of a loss of superior visual field and desire surgical repair. Many third party payers require documentation of the visual disability before they

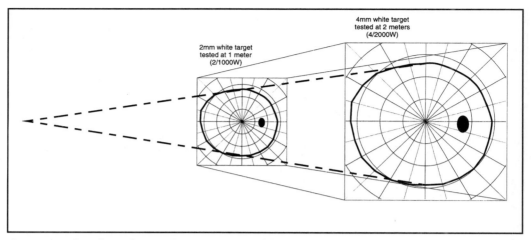

Figure 6-4. The effect of target distance on size of field.

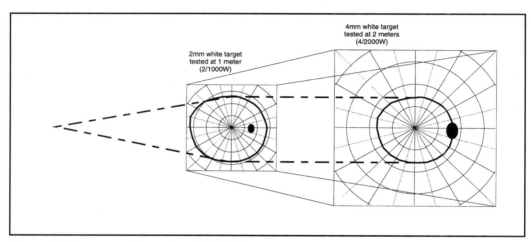

Figure 6-5. Non-expanding or "tunnel field."

will reimburse for the surgery. To satisfy this requirement, visual field testing is necessary.

The method used is essentially the same as measuring any patient's visual field. The technique selected must evaluate the superior visual field, but automated perimetry, Goldmann perimetry, and tangent screen testing can all suffice. The program used in automated perimetry must test beyond 15° to 20° in order to detect abnormalities in the field due to ptosis; the Humphrey Field Analyzer program 30-2 and the Octopus program 32 are both acceptable routines.

The patient is tested in the usual manner for the technique selected. Usually the result will show constriction or depression in the superior visual field. The patient's eyelids or brows are then supported with tape to temporarily relieve the ptosis. The test is then repeated and the results compared. The taping must be done in such a fashion as to allow the patient to blink and prevent the cornea from drying out. If the patient's blink is impaired from the tape, the test should be paused intermittently and the tape removed to allow the patient to blink and restore the tear film. The tape is then replaced and the testing continued. The superior field loss should show improvement when the lid is elevated. An example is provided in Figure 7-14.

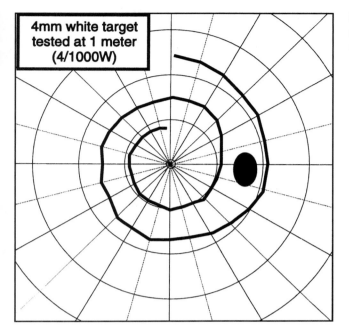

4mm white target
tested at 1 meter
(4/1000W)

Figure 6-6. Spiral visual field commonly found in non-physiologic visual loss.

Binocular Field Testing

Patients with restrictive or paralytic strabismus frequently have double vision in some field(s) of gaze. This double vision, or diplopia, is caused by misalignment of the visual axes of the two eyes. Visual field testing techniques can be used to determine the regions of single and double vision in these patients. Diplopic field testing is best accomplished using the Goldmann or similar kinetic perimeter. A tangent screen can be used if the area of single vision is restricted to the central 20° or so.

For testing with the Goldmann perimeter, the patient is positioned comfortably in the perimeter with the chinrest centered and the corrective lenses properly positioned. In the case of high refractive error (greater than 8 diopters of hyperopia or myopia), contact lenses may be used. Both eyes are left open. A relatively easy-to-see target is presented in the central field. The patient is instructed to *look at the stimulus* and tell if it is single or double. If the patient reports seeing two targets, the stimulus is moved slowly in an attempt to locate a region in which the target appears to be single. (This task is made easier if the perimetrist knows in which direction the patient's eyes appear to be in alignment or where the patient reports to see singly.) Once an area of single vision is determined, the patient is instructed to keep his or her head positioned straight forward in the perimeter, to follow the stimulus as it is moved in the perimeter bowl, and to report as soon as the stimulus becomes double. The stimulus is moved back into the single vision region. The process continues with the stimulus being moved in at least eight directions to determine the size of the area of single vision (in a manner similar to determining the size and shape of a scotoma). Usually only one size stimulus needs to be used. Because the diplopia is gaze-dependent, it is important to be sure the patient's head does not turn to follow the stimulus; only the eyes should rotate. Once the testing is complete, the result is plotted, taking care to clearly indicate which areas represent single and double vision.

Chapter 7

Errors in Visual Field Testing and How to Minimize Them

KEY POINTS

- Proper technique in visual field testing is essential to make sure that any defects detected are the result of disease and not due to an error in the performance of the test.

- Perimeters need to be calibrated on a regular basis to ensure that proper background and stimulus intensity levels are obtained.

- To avoid common errors, particular attention must be directed to the patient's pupil size, refractive error, plus the positioning of the correcting lens.

Introduction

The visual field examination is often very important for the proper diagnosis and management of disorders of the visual system. Proper technique in visual field testing is essential to make sure that any defects are the result of disease and not due to some artifact of the testing procedure (leading to possible incorrect diagnosis and/or inappropriate treatment). This chapter will discuss some of the more common errors and test situations that can give rise to suboptimal results. The examples are real fields encountered in the practices of the authors and are therefore from the Humphrey Field Analyzer (with the exception of Figure 7-9). Similar situations are certainly possible with all other visual field testing techniques.

Machine Calibration

Goldmann Perimeter

In Chapter 4, the importance of calibrating the stimulus intensity and background illumination of the Goldmann perimeter was discussed. One of the advantages of the Goldmann's design is the use of a single bulb to provide both background and stimulus illumination. As long as the machine is set up properly, the ratio of stimulus to background will remain constant, even if the bulb is beginning to fail and the maximum intensity cannot reach 1,000 asb. If the background is not set properly by adjusting the hood on the projector, the proper retinal adaptation is not achieved and the patient's sensitivity will be altered.

A bigger problem arises with regard to standardization and reproducibility. By altering the conditions required for the test, differences in results become difficult to explain. Do the isopters appear abnormal because the patient has disease, or was the patient's sensitivity reduced because the background was too bright and the retina was bleached? More importantly, are changes over time due to a worsening of the disease or to variations in the machine calibration? If visual field testing is to be done with the Goldmann perimeter, it is essential to calibrate it properly.

Automated Perimeter

The Humphrey Field Analyzer cannot not be calibrated by the technician. It uses separate bulbs for the stimulus (maximum 10,000 asb) and background (31.5 asb). When the Humphrey perimeter is turned on at the beginning of a day, a series of automatic internal checks begins. The computer memory and software are tested to be sure they are functioning properly. The CRT (cathode ray tube) will display a message that a "RAM" test is being performed. The background illumination in the bowl is measured by the internal light meter, and the projector is tested, both for accuracy of projection and for brightness of the maximum stimulus. A message will be displayed on the CRT if a bulb needs to be replaced. Other fault conditions will result in a message display and instructions.

When the projector bulb is no longer able to project a 10,000 asb stimulus, this does not prevent testing from continuing. The decrease may not make any difference in patients with normal or near normal sensitivity values, but if the actual sensitivities are reduced, the machine may not be capable of generating the required intensity values to test them. This condition can be identified from a threshold test where the patient did not respond to the brightest stimulus available. Under normal circumstances, a point at which no response was obtained is indicated on the printout by a threshold value indicated by " <0." When the projector bulb is no longer able to generate a 10,000 asb stimulus (0 dB attenuation), the printout will show the value in decibels of the maximum stimulus it was able to project as is illustrated in Figure 7-1. Because the maximum stimulus available was 1 dB (or 7,493 asb), and the patient didn't respond to that stimulus, the "<" sign appears on the printout. Should values other than "<0" appear on the printouts, the projector bulb should be changed as soon as possible.

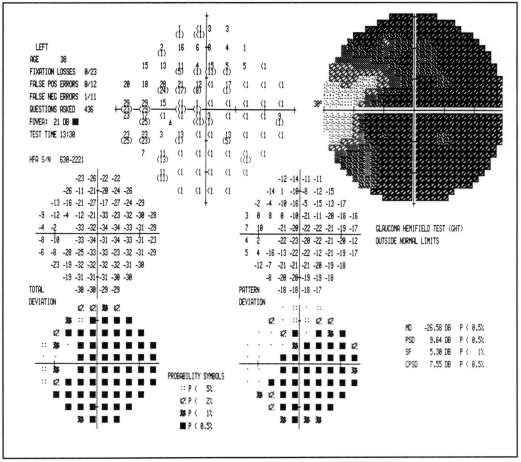

Figure 7-1. Threshold visual field from a patient with severe visual field loss. Note areas with values recorded as "<1," indicating that the projector bulb was incapable of generating a stimulus of 10,000 asb intensity and needed to be changed.

Maintenance of Automated Perimeters

OptA

Most automated perimeters require little maintenance. Be attentive when the machine "boots" because messages that are displayed as the system checks are performed could be missed.

The Humphrey Field Analyzer has proven to be very reliable and the need for repairs minimal. Fortunately, down time has been almost non-existent. Maintenance requirements are also minimal and are outlined in the user manual. Remember when changing the projector bulb not to touch the bulb itself, as this may affect the bulb's life and brightness. Remember to also periodically check the focus of the stimulus as outlined in the manual.

Above all else, routinely back up patient data. If using a hard drive system, keep duplicate copies on floppy disks and back up weekly with the streamer tape. If using the floppy drive system, make sure that two copies of every test are made.

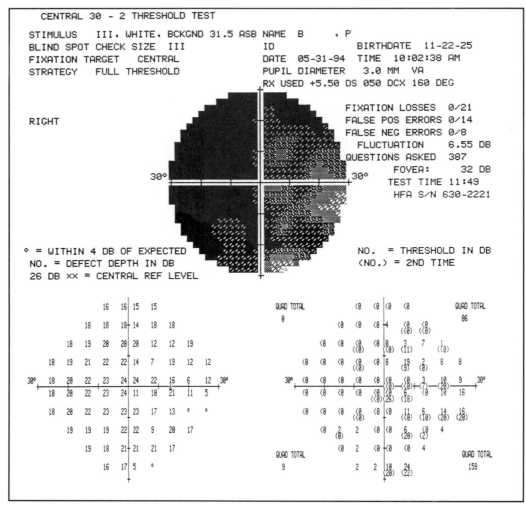

Figure 7-2. Advanced loss in a patient with severe optic nerve damage. The nature of the loss cannot be discerned because the entire field is so depressed.

Stimulus Selection

If proper test techniques are used with the Goldmann perimeter as discussed in Chapter 4, proper stimulus selection will be based on threshold techniques. Rather than testing with an empiric stimulus, the size and intensity will be determined prior to plotting the isopters by actually measuring threshold at a point in the visual field expected to have remaining sensitivity, even in patients with end-stage disease. A stimulus slightly brighter or larger will then be used to map the initial isopter, with reasonable certainty that it will elicit sufficient responses from the patient in order to plot the isopter.

Difficulties may arise in automated perimetry, particularly with threshold testing in patients with low sensitivity levels. Threshold is determined at each test point by varying the stimulus intensity until the appropriate responses have been elicited, keeping the stimulus size constant. The default stimulus on the Humphrey Field Analyzer is equivalent to the Goldmann size III. Patients with far-advanced disease may not have sufficient sensitivity remaining in their visual field to respond even to the brightest stimuli when the size is fixed at III. An example is given in Figure 7-2. The entire visual field in Figure 7-2 demonstrates

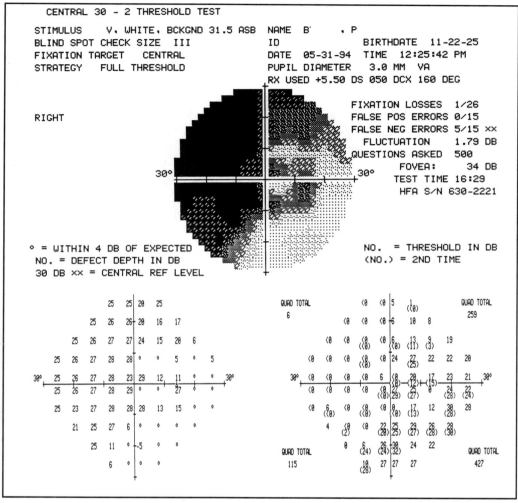

Figure 7-3. The visual field from the same patient as Figure 7-2 after repeating the examination with a larger stimulus (V). The double-arcuate nature of the loss is revealed.

significant depression to the stimulus size III, failing to respond at most of the test points even at 10,000 asb intensity (indicated by "<0" on the value table at the lower right grid on the printout). The pattern of this loss cannot be determined, and a diagnosis could not be made based on the visual field information. Sometimes this degree of depression results from media opacities such as cataract, or may be the result of advanced glaucoma or other optic nerve disease. The technician should be aware when a patient is not pushing the response button. After determining that the patient is awake, alert, and understands how to perform the test, the technician should conclude that the stimulus is not big enough to be seen. The test should then be stopped and restarted after changing to a larger size. Usually, the size III would be changed to the V, which should result in the equivalent of increasing the relative intensity of the stimuli by a factor of 10. Such a change in stimulus size "amplifies" the remaining visual field and may result in useful data. Figure 7-3 shows the visual field of the patient shown in Figure 7-2 when retested with a stimulus size V. The double arcuate nature of this patient's loss is apparent, indicating that the loss is optic nerve based.

Correcting Lens Errors

One of the greatest sources of error in visual field testing may be the correcting lens. Errors can arise from incorrect power and also from incorrect placement of the lens.

Incorrect Lens Power

In order for the patient to perceive the smallest, dimmest stimulus that will be near threshold for the point being tested, the bowl must be in focus. If the projected stimulus is not in focus, it will have to be made larger or brighter to elicit a response, making the measured field look worse than it really is. Proper lens selection is based on: 1) the current distance refractometric measurement (taking into consideration the effect of dilating the pupil, if necessary); 2) the accommodative state of the eye (mostly determined by age, but also taking aphakia/pseudophakia and dilation into consideration); and 3) the size of the bowl (smaller bowls require larger adds). The proper method for determining the correcting lens power has been discussed in the sections on Goldmann perimetry and automated perimetry.

Figure 7-4 illustrates one common power problem—using the proper distance lens but forgetting to include the appropriate addition for the test distance. No add was used, and this 62-year-old patient had an accommodative requirement of +3.00 diopters for the test distance. The under correction resulted in apparent diffuse loss of sensitivity (indicated by mean deviation or MD in excess of -6 dB).

An example of a lens error based on an incorrect distance prescription is shown in Figure 7-5. The patient was tested with +4.75 sphere, based on a distance measurement of +2.25. The field shows diffuse depression with a mean defect of -7.19 dB. In actuality, the distance refraction was the spherical equivalent of -0.75. The patient was tested the next day with the proper lens (+1.75 sphere) and the resultant field is shown in Figure 7-6. The properly tested field shows mild nasal loss and a mean deviation of -0.77 dB, an across the board improvement of more than 6 dB.

Figure 7-7 is a series of examinations over time of an eye with a refractive error of approximately -4.00 sphere for distance. The patient required a +3.00 add. In the second examination of the series, the technician mistook the distance prescription for +4.00, and thus tested the eye with a +7.00 (an 8 diopter error from the -1.00 that should have been used). This resulted in a diffuse change from the first examination of more than 11 dB! Repeating the test 2 days later with the proper lens power (last field in the series) showed that there was no change from the first examination.

The use of foveal threshold as an indicator of possible lens power errors was discussed in Chapter 5.

Correcting Lens Position

Make a circle with the thumb and forefinger of your right hand. Close your left eye, and look through the circle with your right eye with your hand held as close to your eye as possible. Now slowly move your hand away from your eye to a distance of about 1 to 1.5 inches. As you do this, you will note that a portion of your visual field is blocked out by the circle made by your fingers.

You have just reproduced the ring scotoma that may be seen when the correcting lens used for the visual field test is improperly positioned too far from the patient's eye. The edge of the lens or the lens holder is responsible for the defect. Similarly, if the patient is positioned so that the lens holder is too high, an inferior visual field defect that respects the horizontal midline may be created, resembling a glaucomatous field loss. This defect may be distinguished by its characteristic shape (corresponding to the shape of the lens holder), its lack of connection to the blind spot, and its disappearance when the lens is positioned properly. Defects caused by incorrect lens position are more common in patients requiring significant hyperopic correction. Figure 7-8 is the classic rim artifact corresponding precisely to the shape of the correcting lens holder as found on automated perimetry. Figure 7-9 is a Goldmann field where a wide-rimmed lens was used.

The patient in Figure 7-10 sought a second opinion after being started on glaucoma medications based on the illustrated visual field. Her optic nerve was completely normal, and her intraocular pressure (IOP)

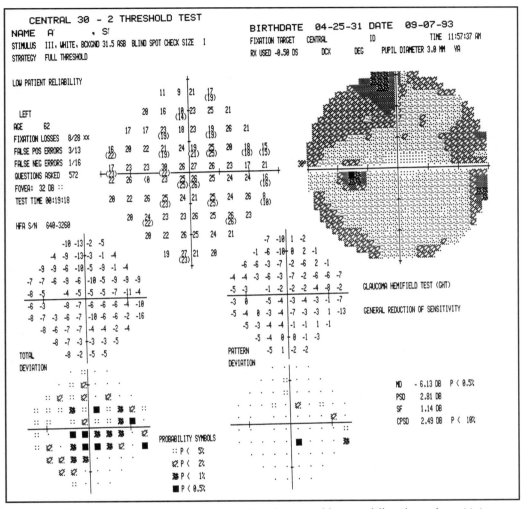

Figure 7-4. Patient tested with correct distance lens but no add. Note diffuse loss of sensitivity.

was 12 mm Hg following cessation of therapy. Her real visual field, performed with the lens in the correct position, is shown in Figure 7-11.

Defects attributed to incorrect positioning of the correcting lens are avoidable with proper positioning of the patient and correct placement of the lens and lens holder. Monitoring throughout the examination is essential, because if the patient's head drifts away from the headrest, the lens will be too far from the eye and these defects will appear. Proper positioning at the start of the test does not necessarily guarantee that the patient will remain in place for the entire examination. The technician should periodically check the patient's head position during the examination and make any necessary adjustments.

Testing Errors Arising from Incorrect Examination Preparation

Set-up Errors on the Humphrey Field Analyzer

The Humphrey Field Analyzer, if equipped with the proper analytical software such as STATPAC or

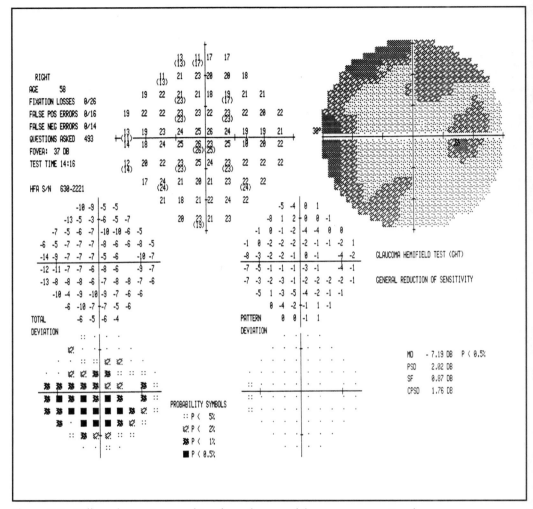

Figure 7-5. Diffuse depression resulting from the use of the wrong correcting lens.

STATPAC II, has the capability of performing statistical analysis of patients' visual fields to determine abnormalities of single fields as well as changes over time. The basis of the comparison is stored data containing normal threshold values derived from examining a large population of disease-free subjects. The database is constructed in such a way that each patient is compared to a peer group of the same age. Entering the correct birth date when the machine is set up for an examination is thus essential to tell STATPAC how old the patient is for comparison to the correct age-matched normal population. Figure 7-12 is an example of a test performed with the patient's birth date entered with the correct month and day, but with the test year entered in lieu of the correct birth year. The machine does not recognize that the birth date entered for the examination is *after* the date of the exam! It does recognize the year (entered as *94*) and assumes that it is *1894*, thus making the patient 100 years old. The patient is then compared to an age-matched population of 100-year-olds and appears to have a mean deviation of -1.86 dB. In reality, the patient was born in 1954, and the printout with the birth date corrected appears in Figure 7-13. Compared to 40-year-olds, the mean deviation is -6.51. Comparing a patient to an older population will make the deviations appear smaller, because the comparison threshold values are lower. Care must be taken when entering the patient information in the machine to avoid this sort of error.

It is also important to enter the patient's name the same way every time. Any alteration will cause a fail-

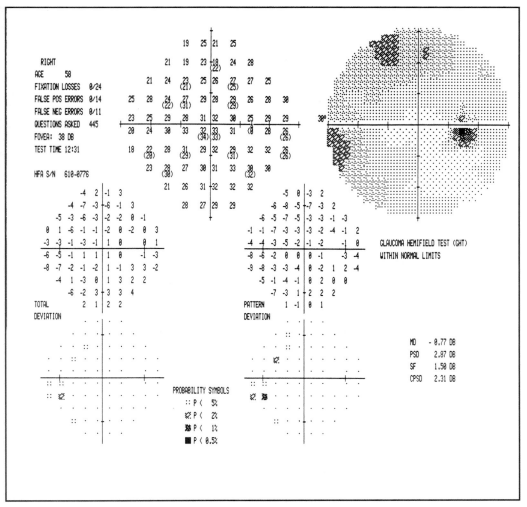

Figure 7-6. Improvement in the visual field when the proper lens was used (same patient as Figure 7-5).

ure to find all of the patient's examinations for overview, change, or STATPAC analysis. Joe Smith, Joseph Smith, and Joe E. Smith are all different patients as far as the machine is concerned. The later versions of the operating software for the perimeter allow the technician to recall patient data from disk files. This option assures that there will be no variations in the patient's name or birth date.

Positioning Errors

The patient must be properly positioned for an examination, without undue distraction. The patient should be seated comfortably on a reasonably soft chair with the neck, shoulders, and arms relaxed. The machine should be at such a height that the patient's forehead is in contact with the headrest when the chin is placed into the chinrest, with no tendency to fall back. Proper patient positioning was discussed in Chapter 5 and illustrated in Figures 5-19 through 5-24. The correcting lens holder artifact illustrated in Figure 7-8 resulted from the patient being positioned too low relative to the machine. She could not keep her head against the headrest and drifted back too far from the lens, resulting in the illustrated defect. The best way to minimize errors is simply to talk to the patient: ask if the bowl is in focus and if he or she is comfortable. The answers can help the technician take the proper action to fix the problems before the test progresses too far.

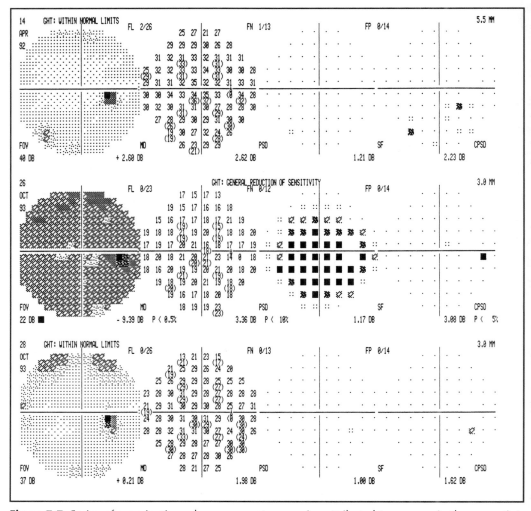

Figure 7-7. Series of examinations show apparent worsening attributed to an error in the correcting lens used in the second examination. Repeat testing with the correct lens in the third examination shows that there was no change from the first exam.

Artifactual Loss

Not all defects seen on a perimetric test are due to disease. The identification of visual field defects due to disease requires that defects from other causes be excluded. Human factors, both on the part of the patient as well as the examiner, influence the performance and results of the test and may give rise to depressions which may be misinterpreted. Artifact in visual field testing may be defined as apparent visual field loss which is not due to any malfunction of the visual system. One of the hallmarks of artifact in the visual field is its lack of correlation to known disease processes. The most commonly seen artifactual losses are due to the correcting lens, eyelids and brows, and inadequate pupil size.

Correcting Lens Artifact

Errors attributable to incorrect lens power and positioning have been discussed.

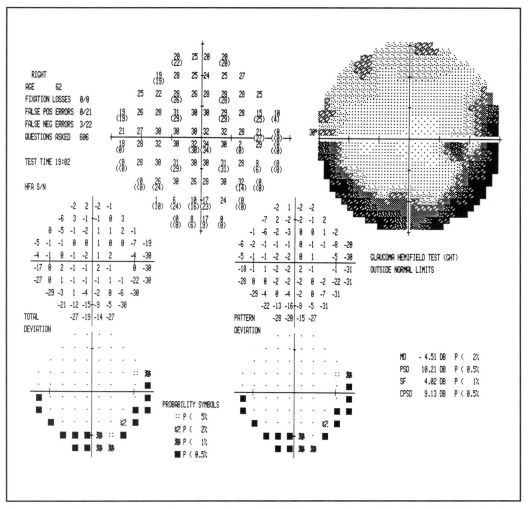

Figure 7-8. The classic artifact due to blockage of the inferior portion of the visual field by the lens holder.

Eyelids and Brows

The anatomy of the patient's face and orbit may, on occasion, give rise to visual field defects misidentified as being due to glaucoma. Patients with prominent superior orbital ridges will often manifest superior visual field depressions which may appear to be a superior arcuate scotoma. This type of defect can be properly identified by its lack of connection to the horizontal midline and the blind spot, as well as by correlation with the appearance of the patient. Ptotic (drooping) upper eyelids may give rise to similarly appearing defects. When any doubt exists as to the cause of such defects, it might be prudent to repeat the examination with the lid taped up or with the patient's head tilted back from the headrest in order to roll the eye down. Taping is preferred, because rolling the eye down may result in further lowering of the upper lid.

The patient shown in Figure 7-14 underwent testing twice in the right eye on the same day. The first visual field, performed at 8:30 am, shows basically no defect. The repeat examination at 9:30 am shows a dense superior defect that does not connect to the blind spot. The defect in the second visual field is due to considerable drooping of the upper lid and excess lid skin. (The first field was performed with the lid taped

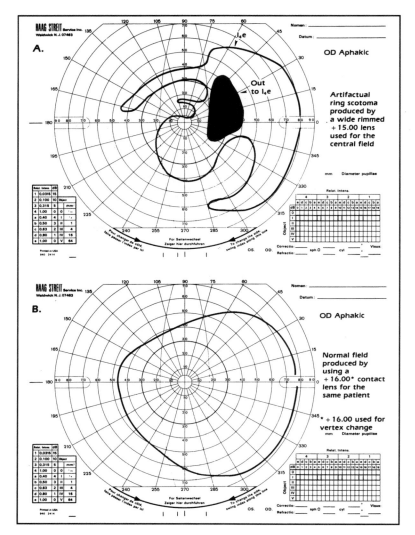

Figure 7-9. (A) Artifactual ring scotoma produced by a wide-rimmed +15.00 diopeter lens used to test the central field. (B) Normal field produced by using a +16.00 diopter contact lens to test the field or by removing the lens to test eccentricities from 20 to 90°.

up.) Figure 7-15 is another example. In this case, the eye was fixating improperly, and the downward rotation of the eye caused the upper lid to droop, resulting in a typical upper eyelid artifact.

Artifactual Loss Due to Small Pupils

Strictly speaking, depression due to small pupils is real visual field loss and not artifact, but it should go away if the field is repeated with the pupils dilated. There appears to be a critical size at which pupil size becomes important. In a study involving normal subjects, constriction of the pupil from 6 mm to 2.5 mm resulted in a uniform (with regard to eccentricity) diffuse depression of approximately 2.5 dB. Pupils of less than 2 mm are more likely to exert a significant effect on the overall level of the visual field, particularly if a media opacity is present in the visual axis. It is recommended that pupils of less than 2 mm be dilated (if safe to do so). Remember to check distance refractometry after dilation and to test with the full add (+3.00) for the test distance regardless of the patient's age, because a dilated patient has minimal or no accommodative ability.

Figure 7-16 shows the effect of dilating the pupil in a patient taking pilocarpine. The top examination, performed with the pupil constricted to 1 mm due to pilocarpine, shows mild diffuse depression and a mean deviation of -3.19 dB. The follow-up examination, performed following pupillary dilation (and appropriate

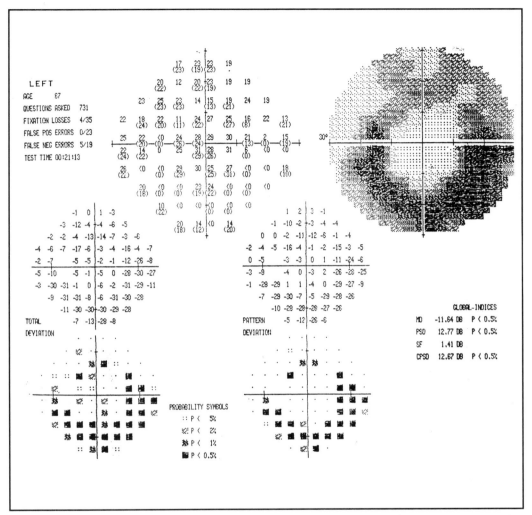

Figure 7-10. Marked decentration of the lens caused this apparent defect. The patient was started on glaucoma therapy based on this visual field despite normal IOP and a normal appearing optic nerve.

post-dilation refractometry), shows no defect and a mean deviation of +0.89 dB, an improvement in mean sensitivity of more than 4 dB. Of course, when dilating the pupils of glaucoma patients, make sure that they do not have occludable angles and make sure to check the IOP following dilation. Some patients, even with open angles, can have significant increases in IOP following dilation. Check with the clinician prior to dilating any patient unless the examination order specifically calls for dilation.

Examination Reliability and Catch Trials

Determination of reliability is essential in the interpretation of visual field examinations. The eyecare professional relies on a number of objective measures of reliability. These measures are incorporated into most automated perimeters, and can be moderated and controlled to a certain degree by an attentive techni-

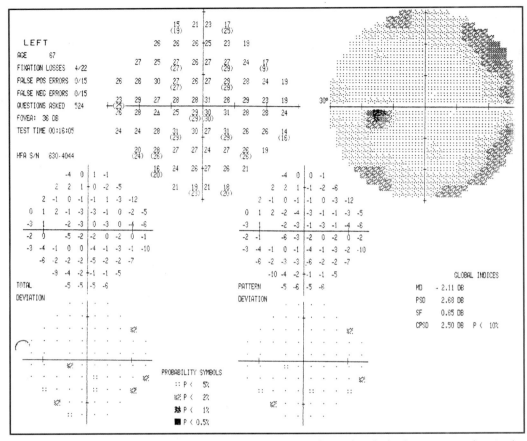

Figure 7-11. Visual field from the patient in Figure 7-10 performed with the lens more or less in the proper position. (Some small lens artifact remains due to the hyperopic refraction required.)

cian. The following discussion pertains to the Humphrey Field Analyzer, but most automated machines use similar techniques.

False Positive Responses

During the performance of any visual field test, the Humphrey Filed Analyzer will periodically move the projector and open the shutter without projecting a stimulus. If the patient pushes the response button to this non-projected stimulus it will be recorded as a false positive response and the machine will beep to alert the technician. A running tally of false responses is shown in the lower right-hand corner of the video display. At each occurrence of a false positive response, the technician should remind the patient to push the button only when a light is seen. Most patients will have some false positive responses during the test, and a rate up to 20% may be considered acceptable. If the patient's rate exceeds 33%, the printout will indicate so by printing "XX" next to the rate. ("XX" next to any of the indices is considered unacceptable by the machine and indicates unreliability.) A high rate of false positives may indicate a patient who is "button-happy." A high rate may occur when the patient does not understand the test or is anxious and concerned with seeing all the lights in order not to be labeled "blind." False positive responses can also occur if the patient learns to respond to the machine noise instead of the light. It is easy to get into the rhythm of the whir of the translation motors and then the click of the shutter opening, usually followed by a light. The

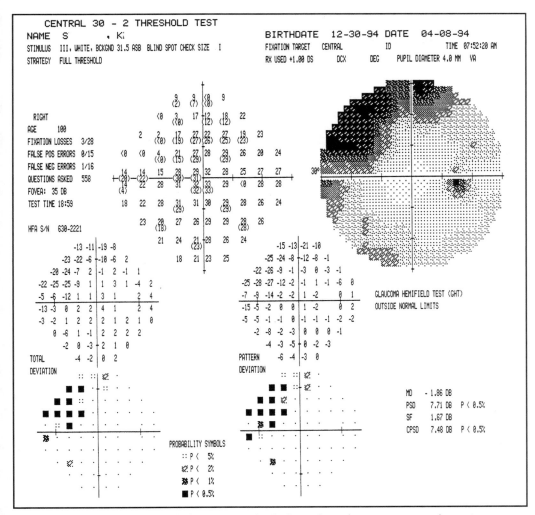

Figure 7-12. Test performed with the incorrect birth date. The software compares the patient to a much older population, making the field look better than it really is. Note the mean deviation is not labeled as abnormal.

cycle may be completed by the button push even if no light was seen, resulting in a false positive response. Later models of the Humphrey Field Analyzer have attempted to limit machine noise by using a "quiet board," but this does not totally eliminate the noises. Some patients still appear to respond to the noise rather than the light. A high false positive rate makes the measured field look better than it really is. In general, a high false positive response rate is the best indication of unreliability, and, unlike the other reliability measures, has no other meaning except that of unreliability.

High false positive responses may affect the field in a number of ways. Sporadic false positive responses, scattered over the field, may give rise to areas of falsely high sensitivity, the "white scotoma." Figure 7-17 is an example of an unreliable visual field showing 7/16 false positive responses (44%). The graytone printout shows multiple white scotomata, corresponding to areas of abnormally high sensitivity. The circled test points in the figure show threshold values that are impossible; the stimulus intensities would be too dim to be seen even by the most sensitive retina under the best test conditions. Because the patient was pushing the button when he really wasn't seeing the lights, the machine kept making the stimuli dimmer until the

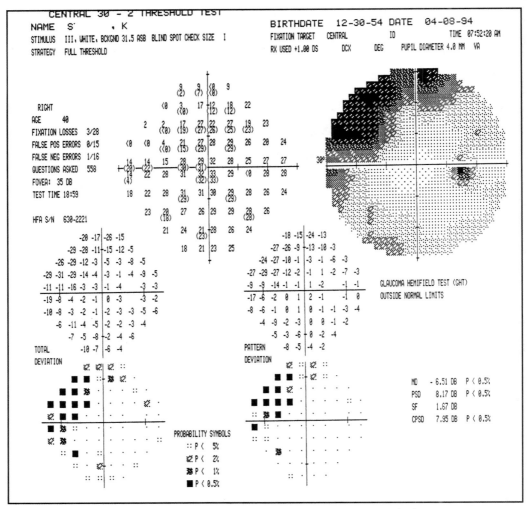

Figure 7-13. Same examination as Figure 7-12 with the birth date corrected. The patient is now compared to the appropriate age-matched normals. Mean deviation is now significantly abnormal.

patient stopped responding. This field is unreliable and must be repeated if it is to have any clinical usefulness.

Figure 7-18 is a more extreme example, showing 90% false positive catch trials, and Figure 7-19 is the ultimate in false positive responses—100%! Almost every point in the field shows a value in excess of 60 dB (the dimmest stimuli available on the Humphrey Field Analyzer)—values which are undetectable by the human visual system. These patients need careful reinstruction and retesting. The technician should be monitoring for such responses and should never allow an examination to proceed if the patient continues making false responses. It is the job of the technician administering the test to find out what the problem is (whether it is a matter of comprehension, anxiety, discomfort, inability to focus inside the bowl, or whatever), correct it, and then allow the exam to conclude. The computer addage "garbage in, garbage out" also applies to automated perimetry, and the technician's job is to help keep the "garbage in" to a minimum.

False Negative Responses

As the test proceeds, the machine identifies areas in which the patient has vision, ie, some points at

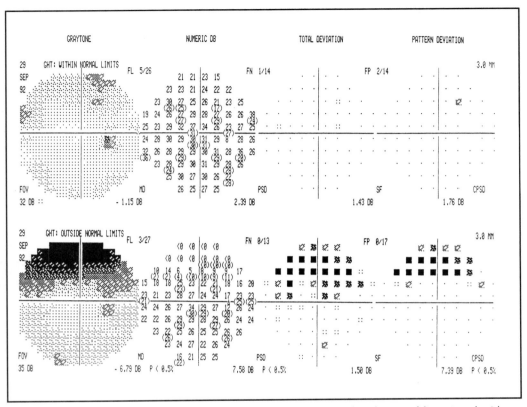

Figure 7-14. Visual field from a patient with upper lid ptosis, tested with (top of figure) and without (bottom of figure) taping of the upper lid.

which threshold measurements were obtainable. During the course of the examination, the machine will come back to a seeing area and project the brightest available stimulus (10,000 asb). Failure to respond to the brightest stimulus in an area previously determined to have some sensitivity is a false negative response. As with false positives, a beep sounds with each occurrence and a tally is kept on the screen. High false negatives may indicate lack of attentiveness, fatigue, or "hypnosis." Some patients may even fall asleep toward the end of a long test. The technician should be alert to this and talk to the patient after each false negative response, pausing the test if necessary to allow rest. In general, a high false negative rate (greater than 20%, although the machine defaults to 33%) makes the field look worse than it really is. However, small (undetectable) shifts in fixation in a patient with marked visual field loss may result in projection of stimuli into a scotoma when it previously was in the "seeing" field. This results in a high false negative rate. Fields should not be considered unreliable solely based on the false negative response rate, however, particularly if there is a great deal of pathology.

The patient in Figure 7-20 has far advanced glaucomatous optic nerve damage. He exhibits 50% false negative responses, which can be attributed to small shifts in fixation. With only very small areas of reasonable sensitivity remaining (circled points), it does not take much movement for a projected stimulus to land in a blind area. This field is otherwise acceptable and is consistent with severe damage.

The visual field in Figure 7-21 shows 100% false negative responses and most likely indicates that the patient did not know what to do. Figure 7-19 is her second attempt after being instructed to push the button when she thought she saw a light.

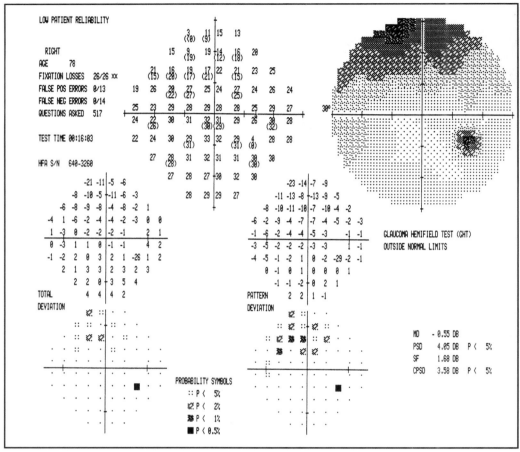

Figure 7-15. One hundred percent fixation losses resulting from fixation on the lower target instead of the center. The eye is rotated down, causing the upper lid to droop so an artifactual defect due to the upper lid is also present.

Fixation Losses

The Humphrey Field Analyzer has the capability of monitoring the fixation behavior of the patient and determining if fixation losses have occurred. The technique used is the Heijl-Krakau method. At the beginning of each test, the machine will locate the blind spot by serially presenting suprathreshold stimuli around the presumed blind spot until the boundaries are located. A small triangle will appear on the video display and the printout, indicating the location of the blind spot. During the test itself, stimuli are periodically projected into the center of the mapped blind spot. A patient response to this stimulus presentation is presumed to have resulted from a shift of fixation. A running tally of fixation losses and trials is displayed on the video monitor during the test, with a beep at each occurrence to allow the technician to remind the patient about fixating steadily on the target. Twenty percent fixation losses is considered unreliable. Although a high fixation loss rate may indicate poor fixation behavior and unreliability, fixation deviations should also be monitored by the technician through the telescope or video eye monitor. It is possible that in some patients the blind spot is smaller than the area of the stimulus used to check for fixation losses, and thus the projected stimulus would fall on seeing retina. A false fixation loss would then be recorded as an actual loss. Incorrect location of the blind spot or a shift in the patient's position after the test has started may give a high fixation loss rate despite good fixation behavior. High false positives may also result in a high fixation loss rate,

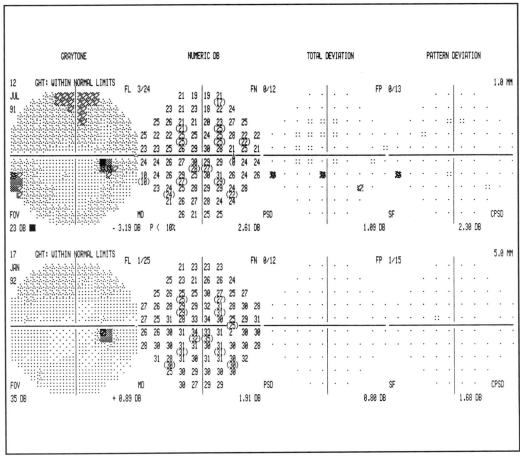

Figure 7-16. Effect of pupillary dilation on the visual field. Note the decrease in mean deviation (MD) from -3.19 dB to +0.89 dB when the pupil was dilated from 1.0 mm to 5.0 mm.

because the patient is inappropriately pushing the button anyway. If the observed fixation behavior is better than the fixation loss rate would indicate, consider decreasing the size of the stimulus used for checking fixation losses (this can be done without changing the stimulus size used for the test itself) or pause the test and remap the blind spot. If the technician is to monitor fixation behavior, you can shorten the test time by 10% if you turn the fixation monitor off.

An unusual cause for high fixation losses is shown in Figure 7-15. The blind spot was correctly localized, indicated by the small triangle just below the horizontal meridian 15° temporal to fixation. (Fixation is at the intersection of the vertical and horizontal axes; each hash mark on the axes is 10°.) However, the patient performed the test while fixating on the lower fixation target in the bowl. This served to move his actual blind spot down; this point measured 4 dB and then 0 dB and appears as the black spot below the horizontal on the graytone. Because the machine thought the blind spot was in the area indicated by the triangle but the eye was rotated down, each fixation loss catch trial was in actuality projected onto seeing retina and elicited a response, resulting in a 100% fixation loss rate. Care must be taken in all aspects of test performance to avoid such problems.

Technician Comments

Automated perimetry offers the advantage of decreasing the burden placed on the technician in the per-

OptA

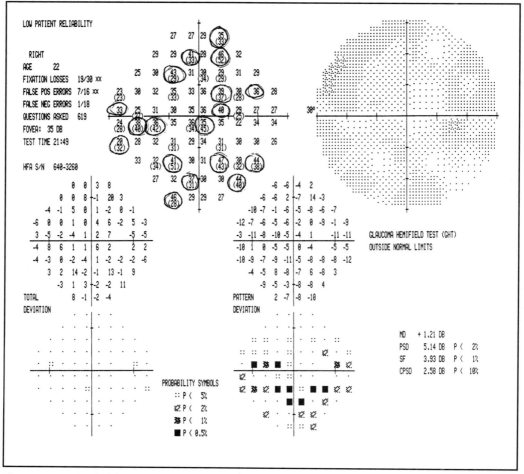

Figure 7-17. Unreliable visual field due to high false positive response rate. Circled points show virtually impossible sensitivity.

formance of visual field testing. However, the role of the technician in assuring the quality of the examination is increased, because the actual performance of the test is left to the computer and the technician is removed from this important interactive phase. The technician must assume an active role in the exam, from the initial greeting of the patient through the printout of the examination results. Patients are human beings, not machines, and may require periodic reminders as to what is expected of them during a perimetric examination. Thus, it is imperative that the technician remain in the room with the patient at all times during the test, not only to supply reinstruction when needed as outlined above, but to act as a source of reassurance and comfort as the patient plods through what is often a difficult task. In this role as instructor, the technician becomes a valuable source of information for the person who interprets the results of the examination. Technicians should be encouraged to write some comments as to the patient's performance during the test, either on the printout or the patient's chart. Comments should include fixation behavior (recorded fixation losses notwithstanding, and mandatory if the fixation monitor is turned off), ability to understand the test procedures, ability to perform the test, fatigue and when it occurred (which eye, tired before the beginning of the examination, etc), cooperation, general attitude, any comments the patient may have made, etc. These comments can be invaluable in interpreting the test results and understanding the other reliability measures as recorded by the machine.

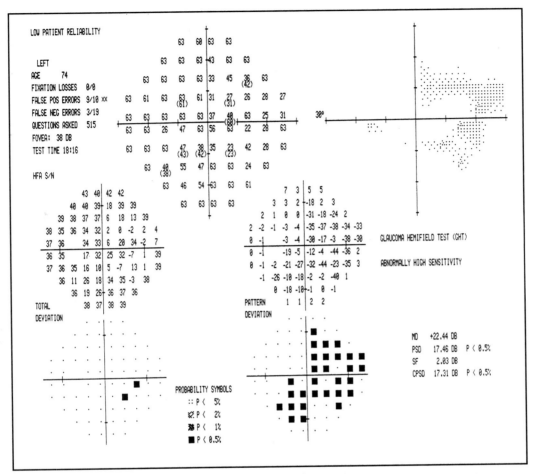

Figure 7-18. An almost white visual field due to 90% false positive response rate.

Maximizing Reliability

It cannot be emphasized enough that proper performance of automated perimetry still requires the presence of a skilled and knowledgeable technician. The technician cannot perform a test without being in the room even though the technician does not have to move the projector and control the shutter. Although the patient received thorough instructions at the beginning of the test, false responses may still occur. The technician should be present to observe the errors as they happen and take proper measures to prevent the next one. Reinstruct the patient to push the button when a light is seen (reducing false negatives), not to push the button unless a light is seen (reducing false positives), and to maintain fixation on the central light (reducing fixation losses). Fixation should be monitored through the video eye monitor or telescope. If the observed fixation behavior is better than the recorded fixation losses would indicate, the technician should remap the blind spot or reduce the check size. Finally, a comment in the medical record as to the patient's fixation behavior may prove useful to the eye care professional for proper interpretation of the examination results.

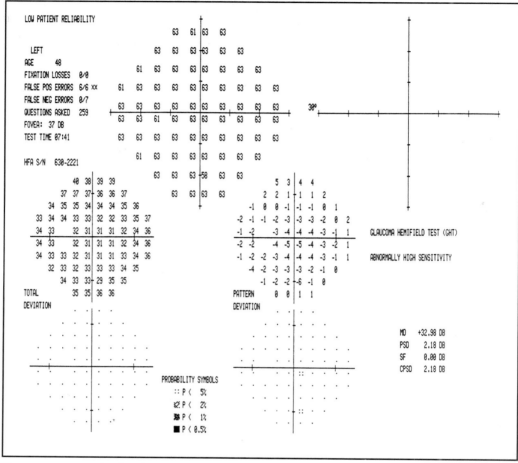

Figure 7-19. Completely white visual field due to 100% false positive response rate. The patient was continuously pushing the response button.

Errors in Test Pattern Selection

Customizing the Test to the Patient

The selection of a visual field test is usually based on what information is sought by the clinician. Often the technician is not given specific guidance as to what test to do; the test performed is usually the "default" examination for the practice setting. A good visual field testing system should be flexible, often requiring decision making on the part of the technician to tailor the test to the ability of the patient. For example, the "standard" visual field test on the Humphrey Field Analyzer is the 30-2 threshold test, which requires about 500 stimulus presentations and 15 to 18 minutes per eye to complete. This may prove to be too much for patients who lack the physical ability or mental power to "survive" the test. This will lead to unreliable data that is not useful for clinical decision making. The technician therefore must alter the test, perhaps changing the pattern to one with less test points like the 24-2, or changing the test strategy to one that determines threshold with less stimulus presentations (such as FASTPAC™). Another alternative might be to abandon threshold testing altogether and switch to a screening test. A patient could be tested with the 76-point screen, which uses the same points as the 30-2 threshold test. Once the patient has been "trained" with a simpler

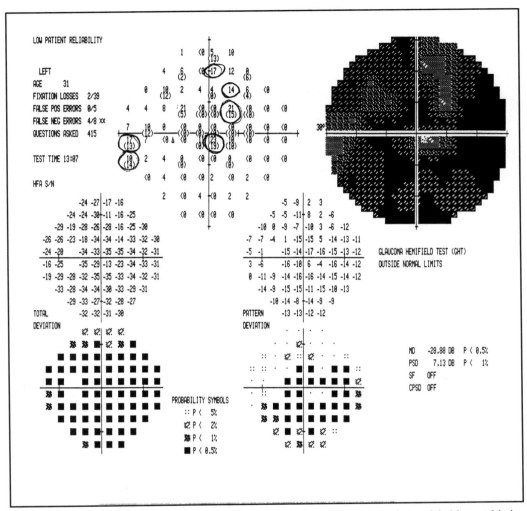

Figure 7-20. The high false negative response rate in this severely damaged visual field most likely resulted from small shifts in fixation, allowing the catch trial stimulus to fall into a non-seeing area. Points remaining with relatively good sensitivity are circled; these are most likely the points used for the false negative catch trials.

type of test, he or she might be able to try the more comprehensive test at a later time.

Test Selection for Patients with End Stage Disease

Changing the stimulus size to "amplify" the remaining visual field in patients with advanced visual field loss has been discussed and illustrated in Figures 7-2 and 7-3. It is difficult, however, for the clinician to evaluate progression of field loss even with the size V stimulus in patients such as those illustrated in this example. Selection of a test that concentrates on the remaining field is often useful. For example, the central 10-2 on the Humphrey Field Analyzer uses a grid of points spaced 2° apart, centered on fixation, offset from the axes by 1°, in the central 10°. This grid gives more data for the remaining visual field than is available with the grids that test farther out. The 10-2 test from the patient illustrated in Figures 7-2 and 7-3 is shown in Figure 7-22. This small central island, tested with stimulus size III, may be followed over time for progression.

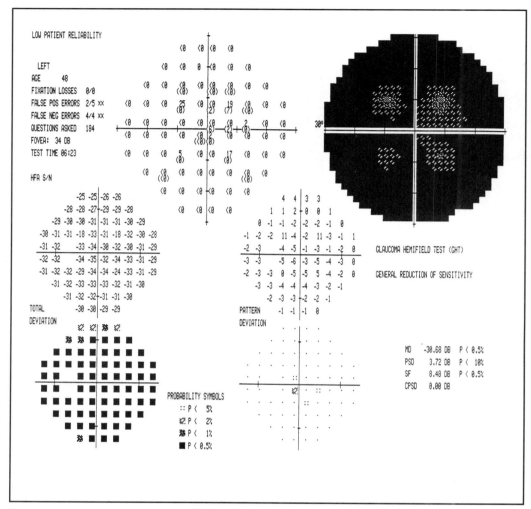

Figure 7-21. One hundred percent false negative responses giving rise to a black visual field. (This is the same patient as Figure 7-18 prior to reinstruction!)

Errors in Defect Detection Due to Use of the Wrong Test Pattern

Test techniques have been discussed in previous chapters. It has been emphasized that the technique employed should be relevant to the patient's diagnosis. For example, the examiner should not spend a lot of time exploring the vertical meridian in a patient with an optic nerve-based disease, such as glaucoma, where the loss is expected to respect the horizontal meridian.

Occasionally the visual field test has to be based on a patient's complaint. Figure 7-23 is the 30-2 from a patient insisting that there was a blind spot in front of his eye. Although the test appeared to be normal, the patient was quite insistent and there was a pigment disturbance in the retina suggestive of some type of injury. He was retested with the 10-2, and the defect became apparent. The defect, illustrated in Figure 7-24, corresponded to the area of pigment disturbance seen in the retina, and was presumed to be a laser injury.

Finally, it is sometimes necessary to keep looking to find a defect that has already been identified if it is not found on the initial try. The patient shown in Figure 7-25 was seen in consultation for glaucoma and had prior Goldmann fields demonstrating a dense superior arcuate scotoma. Her optic nerve was missing rim tissue at the 6 o'clock position, consistent with the Goldmann field. The 30-2 test revealed only mild

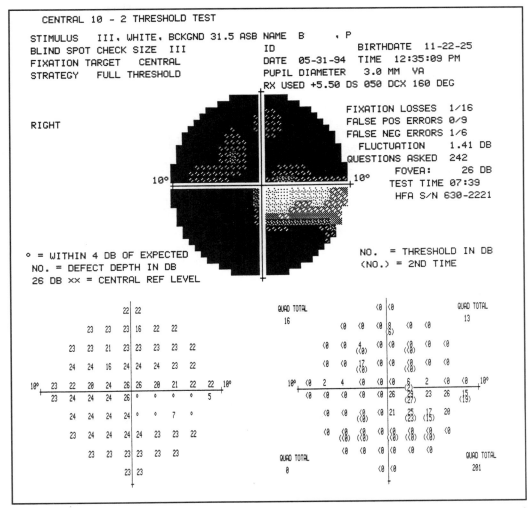

Figure 7-22. The central island of vision remaining in the patient in Figures 7-2 and 7-3 as mapped by the central 10-2 test.

disturbances in the superior hemifield. Suspecting that the scotoma was missed, the test was repeated with the 30-1, Figure 7-26. The 30-1 test points, like those of the 30-2, are separated from each other by 6°. However, the 30-2 test points begin 3° *off* each axis, while those of the 30-1 begin *on* each axis. The points of the two patterns thus interlock, and the scotoma was found on the 30-1, lurking between the test points of the 30-2.

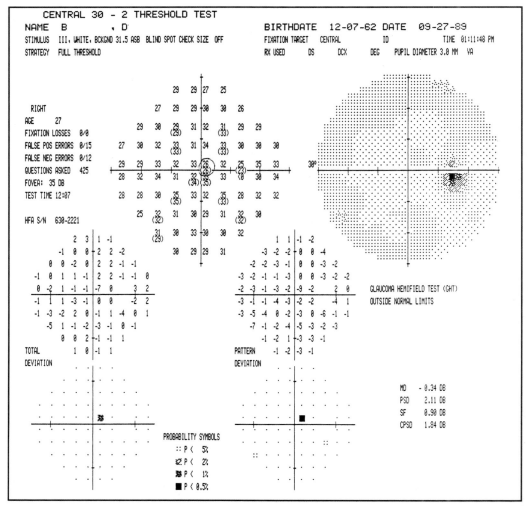

Figure 7-23. Central 30-2 examination from a patient complaining of a subjective blind spot. A small paracentral defect was present (circled).

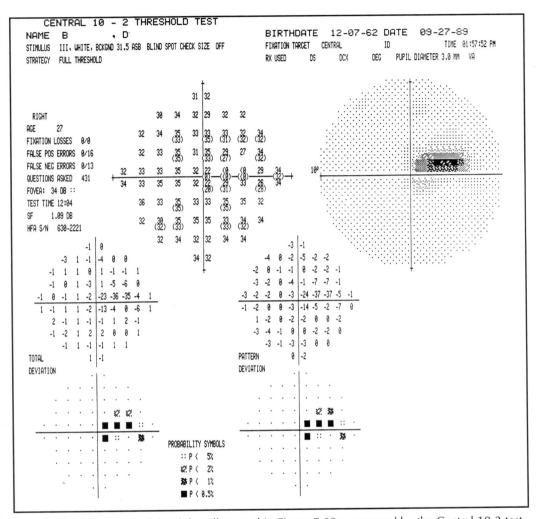

Figure 7-24. "Close-up" of the defect illustrated in Figure 7-23 as mapped by the Central 10-2 test. This was presumed to be a laser injury.

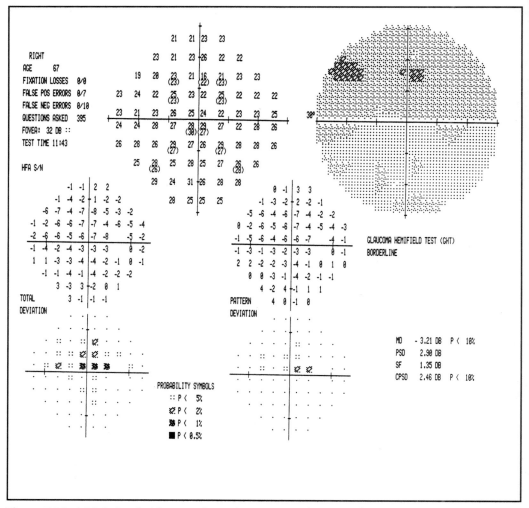

Figure 7-25. A 30-2 threshold test performed on a patient known to have a superior arcuate scotoma demonstrated consistently by Goldmann perimetry. Rim tissue was missing from the optic disc corresponding to the visual field defect.

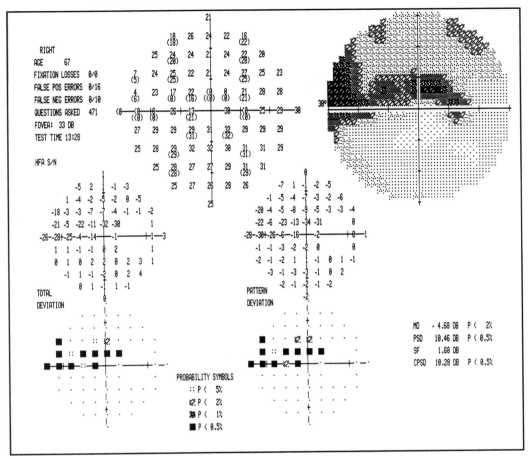

Figure 7-26. A 30-1 test from the same patient illustrated in Figure 7-25. The "missing" scotoma was found between the test points of the 30-2.

Section III

ATLAS OF COMMON VISUAL FIELD DEFECTS

Chapter 8

Visual Field Defects in Glaucoma

KEY POINTS

- Glaucoma is a disorder of the optic nerve, and visual field defects in glaucoma develop as retinal nerve fibers are lost in a characteristic manner.

- Individual defects in glaucoma will respect the horizontal midline, and careful searches should be conducted to identify defects that localize to one side of the horizontal or the other.

- Generalized constriction of the field may occur in the absence of localized defects.

Introduction

Glaucoma is a disease of the optic nerve, and is in reality a group of ocular conditions characterized by progressive loss of the nerve fibers (axons), which make up the optic nerve. The detection of nerve fiber loss and prevention of its development and progression is the ultimate goal in the diagnosis and management of glaucoma. There are two basic modalities of damage to the visual field in glaucoma that may occur singly or together, corresponding to observed patterns of axonal loss. The first is through loss of axons throughout the nerve, with concentric enlargement of the optic cup and thinning of the remaining neuroretinal rim. The entire visual field may be diffusely affected, causing a decrease in threshold for all points, corresponding to a generalized reduction in sensitivity. This is typical of the loss seen early in glaucoma with high intraocular pressure (IOP), and may be due to mechanical compression of axons as they pass through the lamina cribrosa. Secondly, damage may occur in a more focal manner, with enlargement of the cup toward the superior and inferior poles of the disc with loss of portions of the neuroretinal rim, resulting in nerve fiber bundle defects in the visual field. This type of damage has been associated with "low-tension" glaucoma and may be due to decreased blood flow to the nerve.

Patterns of Visual Field Loss in a Single Examination

Generalized Reduction of Sensitivity in Glaucoma

Diffuse depression as the only glaucomatous defect may be detected with threshold testing, especially when statistical analysis is used to compare the patient's results to an age corrected reference population.

The patient illustrated in Figure 8-1 has long-standing open angle glaucoma with recent uncontrolled IOP. He has been on maximum tolerated medical therapy and underwent argon laser trabeculoplasty when his IOP rose into the upper 20s. This visual field demonstrates diffuse depression of the visual field, with a mean defect of -6.50 dB. The glaucoma hemifield test readily identifies the generalized reduction of sensitivity. The test was performed with the appropriate optical correction following dilation of the pupils including the full +3.00 add, and the optical media was clear. Review of the disc photographs showed a gradual increase in the cup-to-disc ratio over time, corresponding to the gradual diffuse loss of sensitivity.

The results of psychophysical tests, such as visual field testing, are subject to a certain degree of variability. This test-retest variability in threshold perimetry is measurable, has known normal values, and has clinical significance. It has been shown that as retinal sensitivity decreases, the variability of threshold in that region increases. It has also been shown that increasing fluctuation may precede the development of a visual field defect, thus giving its measurement particular clinical importance. Figure 8-2 illustrates a patient with post traumatic glaucoma with IOP in the low 30s. The field demonstrates diffuse depression and an eyelid artifact (the globe was enophthalmic due to orbital floor fracture so that the upper lid was ptotic), but more importantly an increased short-term fluctuation value of 3.36, expected in less than 2% of the reference population. The high value is derived from two points in the superior arcuate area (circled)—one showing measurements of 35 and 25 dB and the other 28 and 20 dB. These large differences in repeat measurements (10 dB and 8 dB respectively) point to disturbed portions of the visual field that will most likely go on to develop paracentral and arcuate defects. The short-term fluctuation measurement is very important in evaluating glaucoma patients and glaucoma suspects, particularly because increasing fluctuation may be the earliest sign of glaucomatous optic nerve damage.

Early Focal Loss in Glaucoma

The anatomy of the retinal nerve fiber layer is discussed in Chapter 2. The visual field defects observed in glaucoma result from the loss of axons. The size and shape of these defects is determined by the location

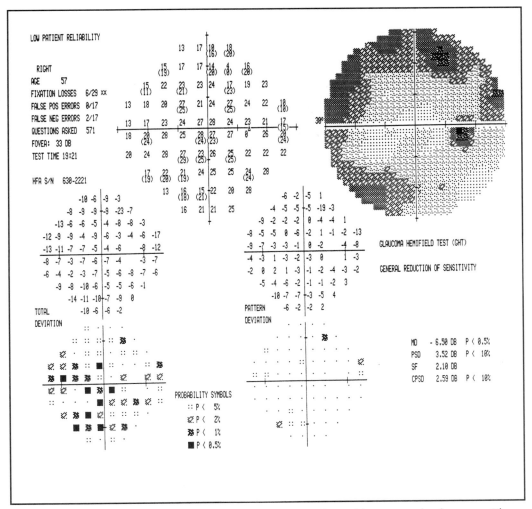

Figure 8-1. An example of diffuse loss of sensitivity in a patient with open angle glaucoma. The patient had clear optical media and was tested with dilated pupils and the appropriate optical correction.

and extent of the nerve fiber loss; loss of arcuate fibers on the temporal side of the disc will result in arcuate defects, and loss of radial fibers on the nasal side will result in wedge-shaped defects. (Of course, due to the optics of the eye, the location of the visual field defect will be reversed superior to inferior and nasal to temporal with respect to the location of the nerve fiber loss. For example, a defect in inferotemporal nerve fibers will result in a superonasal visual field defect.)

Isolated paracentral defects occur as the initial glaucoma defect in about 40% of patients. Other early manifestations of glaucoma damage include arcuate defects, nasal steps, and temporal wedge defects. The patient illustrated in Figure 8-3 shows an isolated defect in the superior paracentral region measuring 22 dB below normal. Note also the wide fluctuation in repeat measurements of this point (13 dB then 0 dB). Untreated IOP was in the upper 20s in this eye.

Figures 8-4 through 8-8 are additional examples of early glaucomatous defects. Defects such as those in Figure 8-5 indicate early damage to the superior pole of the optic nerve and are both parts of the same nerve fiber bundle. If damage continues in this area, these defects will coalesce to form a complete nerve fiber bundle defect.

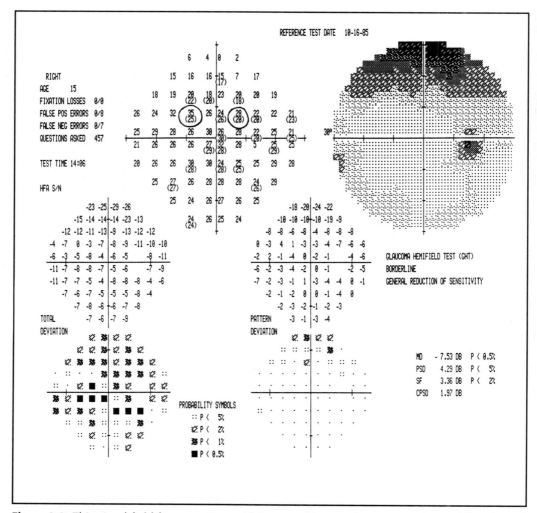

Figure 8-2. This visual field from a patient with increased intraocular pressure shows diffuse loss of sensitivity and an increase in short term fluctuation, indicated by the large spread in repeat threshold measurements in the two circled points. This patient is likely to develop a visual field defect in this disturbed portion of the visual field.

Wedge-shaped defects such as that in Figure 8-8 owe their peculiar shape to the radial orientation of the nerve fibers on the nasal side of the disc. Such defects occur as the initial defects in glaucoma less than 3% of the time.

Advanced Glaucomatous Visual Field Loss

Loss of larger bundles of nerve fibers results in more extensive visual field defects. Figure 8-9 illustrates an almost complete nerve fiber bundle defect resulting from extension of the cup to the inferior pole of the disc and loss of rim at the 6:30 position. Figure 8-10 shows complete nerve fiber bundle defects, greater in the left eye than in the right eye, in a patient with open angle glaucoma and loss of rim tissue inferiorly in both eyes. The patient in Figure 8-11 has moderately advanced glaucoma damage and shows a "double arcu-

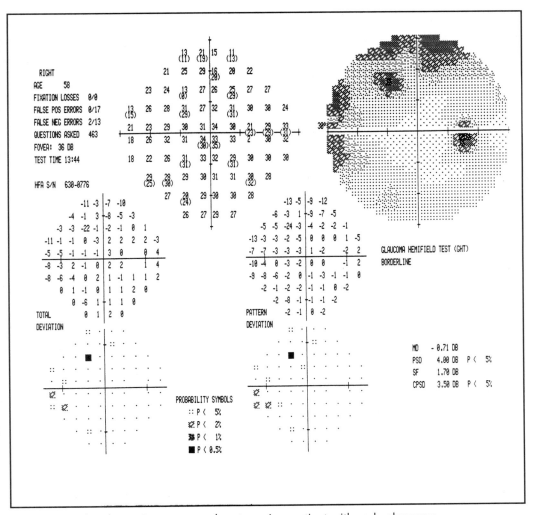

Figure 8-3. Isolated superior paracentral scotoma in a patient with early glaucoma.

ate" scotoma, consisting of superior and inferior nerve fiber bundle defects. Note that the inferior defect is greater than the superior. Just as damage is often asymmetric with respect to the two eyes of a patient, it is often asymmetric with respect to the horizontal midline. As damage continues and visual field loss progresses, an entire hemifield may become involved, resulting in an altitudinal defect, as illustrated in Figure 8-12. This patient has low-tension glaucoma and temporal arteritis. Although she never had an episode of ischemic optic neuropathy, it is possible that this sort of damage is partially caused by poor optic nerve blood flow and ischemia. Figure 8-13 shows far advanced glaucomatous loss in a patient with low-tension glaucoma, with a small central island and temporal field remaining.

Finally, Figure 8-14 is the visual field of a patient with end-stage glaucomatous visual field loss who has reduced central acuity due to the optic neuropathy. This patient has a juvenile onset glaucoma and became symptomatic as his loss extended into his central field. This figure was his visual field on presentation, when IOP was in the 50s. Following filtering surgery and stabilization of his pressure in the low teens, his visual acuity improved from 20/70 to 20/25, and some portions of this field improved.

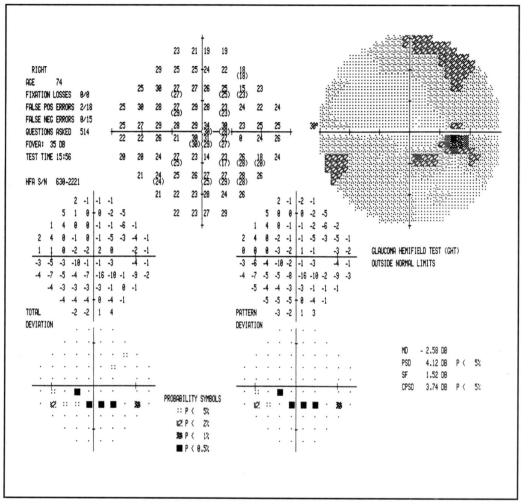

Figure 8-4. Isolated inferior arcuate scotoma without diffuse loss.

Progression of Glaucomatous Visual Field Loss

Uncontrolled glaucoma may show progressive visual field loss in a number of ways as the reserve of nerve fibers is used up and as fibers continue to be lost. Patients with no initial defects may first manifest diffuse loss of sensitivity, increased short-term fluctuation, or begin to develop focal defects. Continued loss may result in further diffuse loss of sensitivity, widening and deepening of existing focal defects as further axons within a bundle become involved, or development of new defects in other portions of the field as new bundles become damaged. Of course, any combination of the above changes may be observed.

Figure 8-15 is an example of the development of diffuse loss of sensitivity over a 7-year period in a man with elevated IOP. Although his pressure had been treated from the beginning, it was uncontrolled at various times during this follow-up period and he required laser treatment. The glaucoma change probability plot shows how he gradually lost sensitivity throughout the field in a manner not expected in the age-corrected reference population of stable glaucoma patients. Note that over this period of time the mean deviation increased from approximately 1 dB to 6.5 dB. This is particularly evident in the graph of mean deviation in the upper right of Figure A. Review of optic disc photographs obtained during this period of time

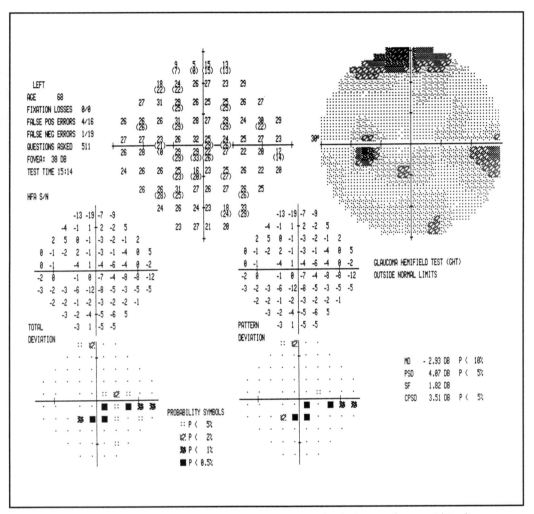

Figure 8-5. Paracentral defects (inferior arcuate scotoma) and inferior nasal step within the same nerve fiber bundle without diffuse loss.

showed a gradual enlargement of the cup to disc ratio, consistent with this diffuse change in the visual field. See Figure 8-1 for the last field in this series.

Fields initially showing defects may later show the development of new defects. Figure 8-16 is a series of fields in a patient with open-angle glaucoma showing completion of an inferior nerve fiber bundle defect as well as the development of new defects in the superior field. Part of the diffuse change in the later fields is due to the development of cataract.

Visual fields may progress by the widening and deepening of single nerve fiber bundle defects. The series of visual fields in Figure 8-17 is from the same patient as Figure 8-9. Initially the field showed mild superonasal loss and then she developed disturbances in the superior arcuate area. These coalesced and extended over time to involve almost the entire bundle of axons and a good portion of the superior field.

The series of visual fields shown in Figure 8-18 was obtained from the fellow eye of the same patient in Figure 8-14. Note the gradual enlargement of the superior nasal step. The IOP on maximum tolerated medical therapy was in the mid-twenties, and he has undergone filtering surgery in this eye.

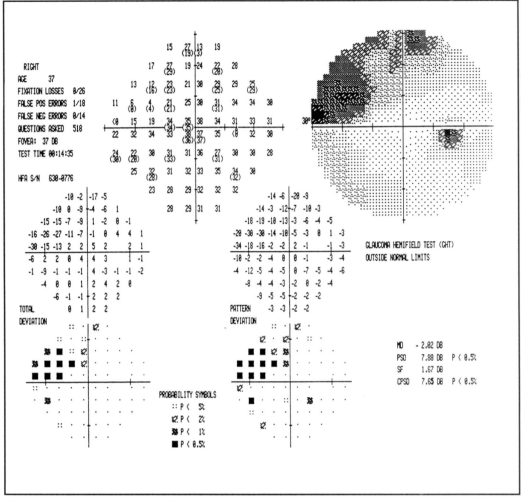

Figure 8-6. Moderately advanced superior nasal step in juvenile glaucoma.

Figure 8-19 is the series of visual fields of the same patient in Figure 8-13. The initial inferior nerve fiber bundle defect has extended, and the patient has developed new defects in the superior hemifield. The statistical software plots the mean deviation over time as a graph (on the top right of the printout in Figure A) and performs statistical tests for significant change over time. This series shows a steady decline of about 0.8 dB per year. This is considered statistically significant.

Finally, Figure 8-20 illustrates the extension of a dense superior nerve fiber bundle defect to a complete altitudinal defect over a 6-year period.

The next series of figures shows glaucomatous fields analyzed with the Goldmann perimeter.

Early nasal steps can occur as a nasal notch (Figure 8-21). The isopter appears continuous above and below the horizontal raphe except for a depression in the region on one side of the 180° meridian. True nasal steps are defined as a difference of 5° between the upper and lower nasal part of the isopter, with associated paracentral scotomas in the same bundle, or a 10° difference across the horizontal raphe as an isolated finding (Figure 8-22). As paracentral scotomas coalesce, they join with the nasal step and break through the isopter border. True baring of the blind spot is usually associated with a

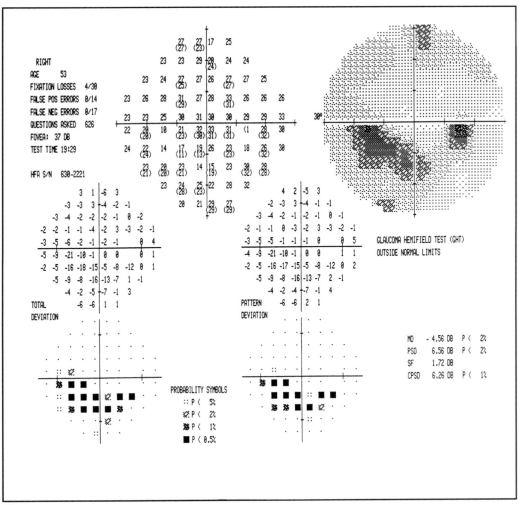

Figure 8-7. Well-developed inferior arcuate scotoma not breaking out to nasal periphery in a patient with end-stage glaucoma in the fellow eye (Reprinted from Garber N. *Visual Field Examination.* Thorofare, NJ: SLACK, Inc; 1988).

nasal step in the Bjerrum area combined with paracentral defects. Extension of the blind spot can occur as an isolated finding, but the perimetrist should look for associated nasal steps. Continuing progression of field loss shows extensive peripheral contraction with a temporal hook around the blind spot (Figure 8-23). Superior or inferior altitudinal defects lead to tunnel vision with 20/20 vision in the central area and a remaining temporal island (Figure 8-24). In advanced glaucoma, the central field is lost leaving a remaining temporal island and a visual acuity of less than 20/400 (Figure 8-25).[1]

Reference

1. Gaber N. *Visual Field Examination.* Thorofare, NJ: SLACK, Inc; 1988.

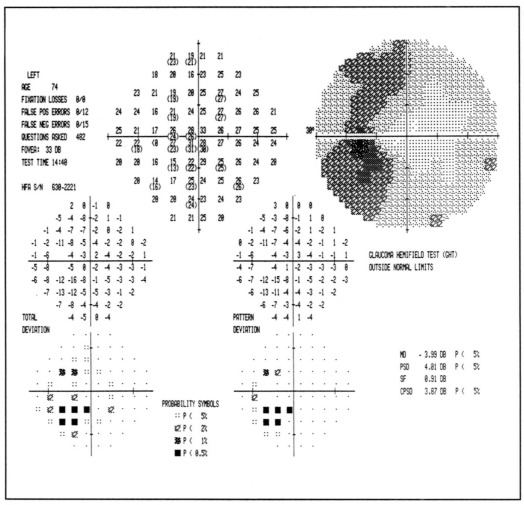

Figure 8-8. Temporal wedge defect in a patient with early glaucoma (Reprinted from Garber N. *Visual Field Examination*. Thorofare, NJ: SLACK, Inc; 1988).

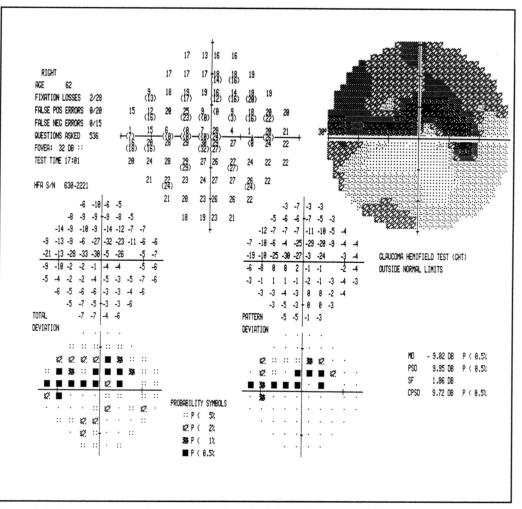

Figure 8-9. Incomplete superior nerve fiber bundle defect, characterized by an arcuate scotoma and superior nasal step (Reprinted from Garber N. *Visual Field Examination*. Thorofare, NJ: SLACK, Inc; 1988).

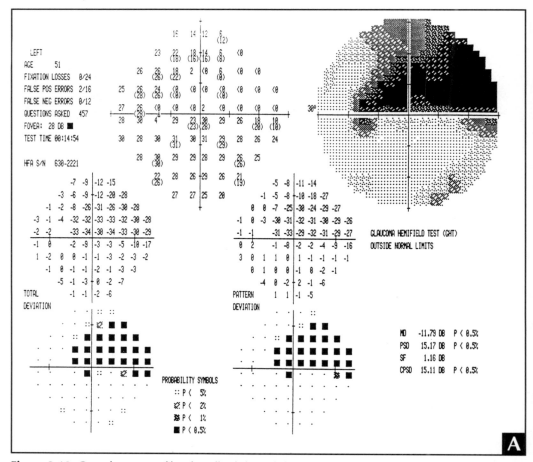

Figure 8-10. Complete nerve fiber bundle defects, left eye (A) greater than right (B), from both eyes of a glaucoma patient (Reprinted from Garber N. *Visual Field Examination*. Thorofare, NJ: SLACK, Inc; 1988).

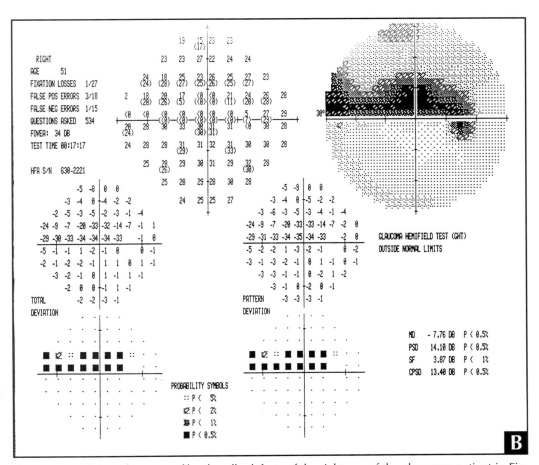

Figure 8-10 (B) Complete nerve fiber bundle defects of the right eye of the glaucoma patient in Figure 8-10 (A) (Reprinted from Garber N. *Visual Field Examination*. Thorofare, NJ: SLACK, Inc; 1988).

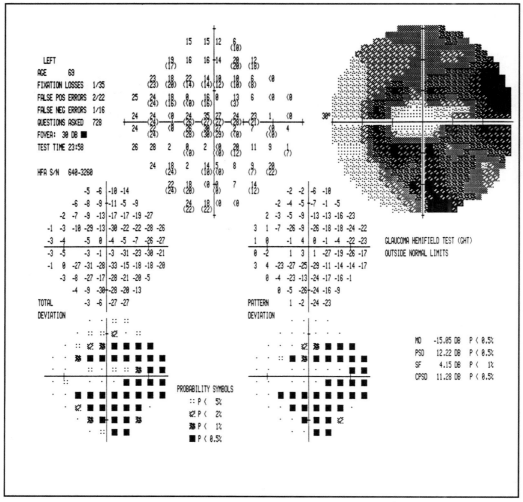

Figure 8-11. The double arcuate scotoma, consisting of nerve fiber bundle defects at both poles of the disc (Reprinted from Garber N. *Visual Field Examination*. Thorofare, NJ: SLACK, Inc; 1988).

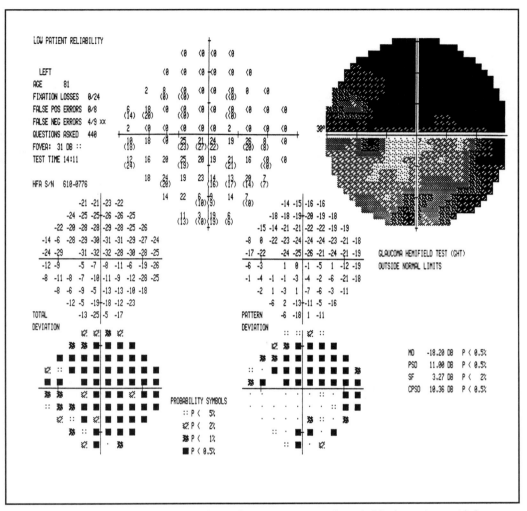

Figure 8-12. An altitudinal defect, involving the entire superior hemifield of a patient with low tension glaucoma and extensive optic nerve damage (Reprinted from Garber N. *Visual Field Examination*. Thorofare, NJ: SLACK, Inc; 1988).

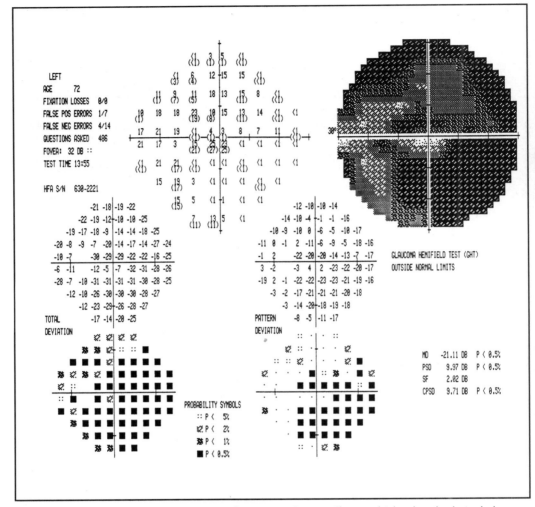

Figure 8-13. Far advanced glaucomatous damage, with a small central island and relatively better temporal sensitivity (Reprinted from Garber N. *Visual Field Examination.* Thorofare, NJ: SLACK, Inc; 1988).

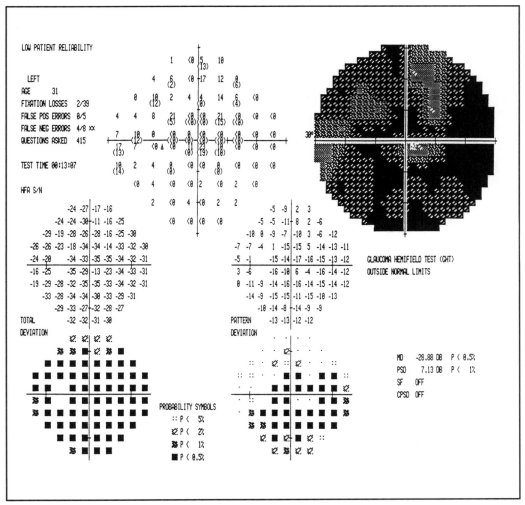

Figure 8-14. End stage visual field in a patient presenting with IOP in excess of 50 mm Hg and far-advanced glaucomatous optic neuropathy (Reprinted from Garber N. *Visual Field Examination.* Thorofare, NJ: SLACK, Inc; 1988).

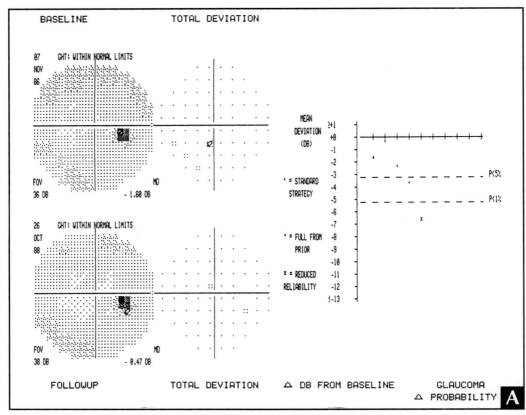

Figure 8-15. Diffuse loss of sensitivity developing over a 7-year period. A. Baseline, B. Follow-up. (Last examination in the series is Figure 8-1) (Reprinted from Garber N. *Visual Field Examination.* Thorofare, NJ: SLACK, Inc; 1988).

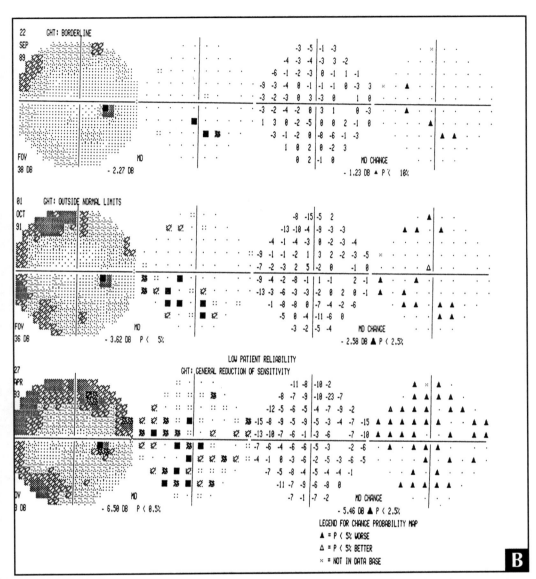

Figure 8-15 (B) Diffuse loss of sensitivity developing over a 7-year period, continued (Reprinted from Garber N. *Visual Field Examination*. Thorofare, NJ: SLACK, Inc; 1988).

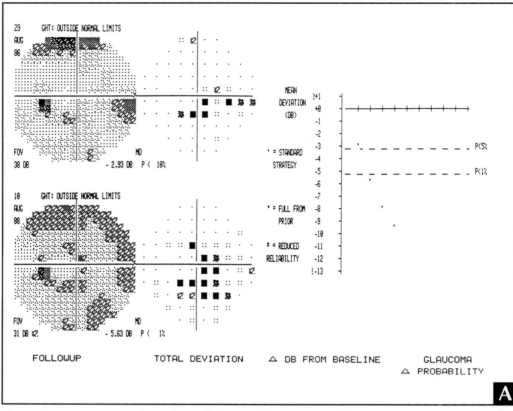

Figure 8-16. Progression of an inferior defect, and development and extension of a superior defect over a 7-year period. A. Baseline, B. Follow-up (Reprinted from Garber N. *Visual Field Examination*. Thorofare, NJ: SLACK, Inc; 1988).

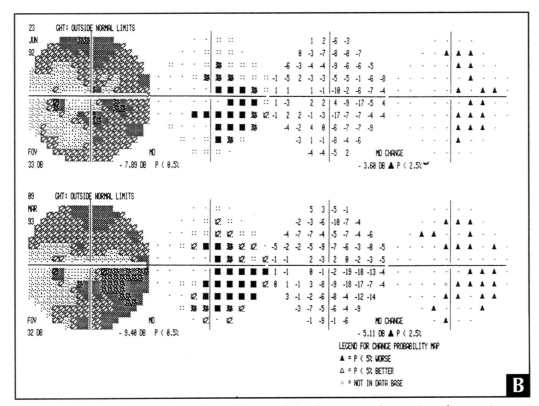

Figure 8-16 (B) Progression of an inferior defect, and development and extension of a superior defect over a 7-year period, continued (Reprinted from Garber N. *Visual Field Examination.* Thorofare, NJ: SLACK, Inc; 1988).

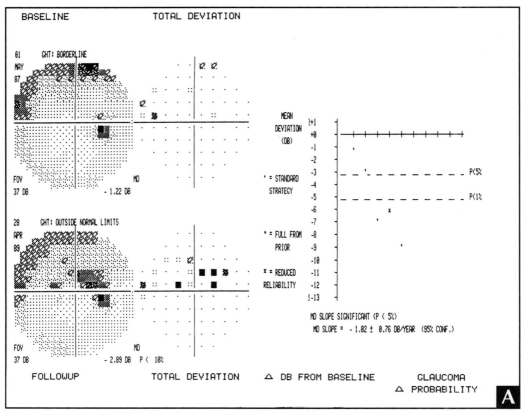

Figure 8-17. Development and extension of a superior defect due to an almost complete nerve fiber bundle defect. A. Baseline, B. Follow-up (The last examination in the series is Figure 8-9) (Reprinted from Garber N. *Visual Field Examination.* Thorofare, NJ: SLACK, Inc; 1988).

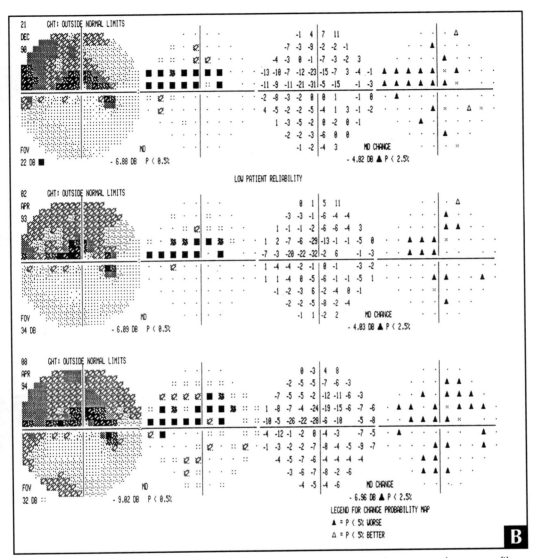

Figure 8-17 (B) Development and extension of a superior defect to an almost complete nerve fiber bundle defect, continued (Reprinted from Garber N. *Visual Field Examination*. Thorofare, NJ: SLACK, Inc; 1988).

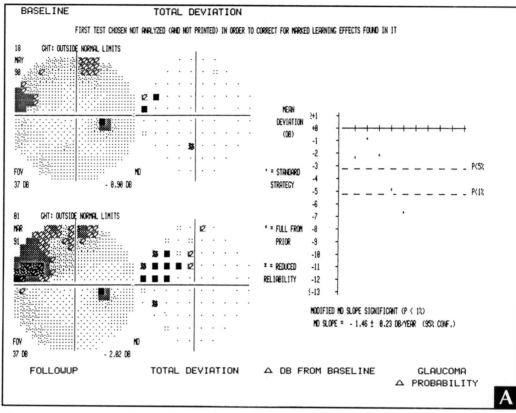

Figure 8-18. Extension of a superior nasal step by widening and broadening. A. Baseline, B. Follow-up (The last examination in the series is Figure 8-14) (Reprinted from Garber N. *Visual Field Examination.* Thorofare, NJ: SLACK, Inc; 1988).

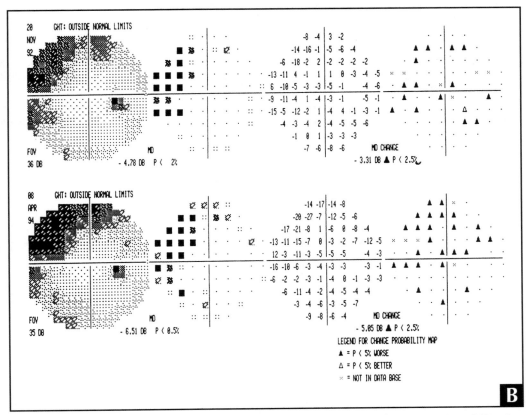

Figure 8-18 (B) Extension of a superior nasal step by widening and broadening, continued (Reprinted from Garber N. *Visual Field Examination.* Thorofare, NJ: SLACK, Inc; 1988).

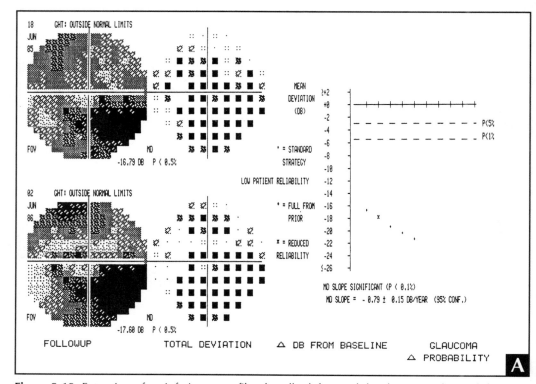

Figure 8-19. Extension of an inferior nerve fiber bundle defect and development of new defects in the superior hemifield. A. Baseline, B. Follow-up (The last examination in the series is Figure 8-13) (Reprinted from Garber N. *Visual Field Examination.* Thorofare, NJ: SLACK, Inc; 1988).

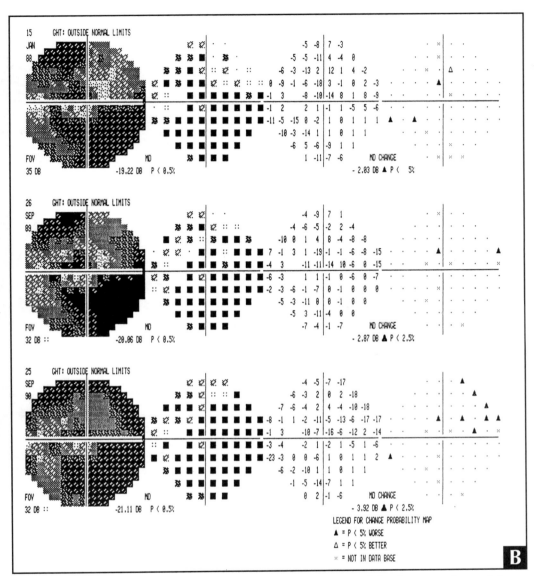

Figure 8-19 (B) Extension of an inferior nerve fiber bundle defect and development of new defects in the superior hemifield, continued (Reprinted from Garber N. *Visual Field Examination.* Thorofare, NJ: SLACK, Inc; 1988).

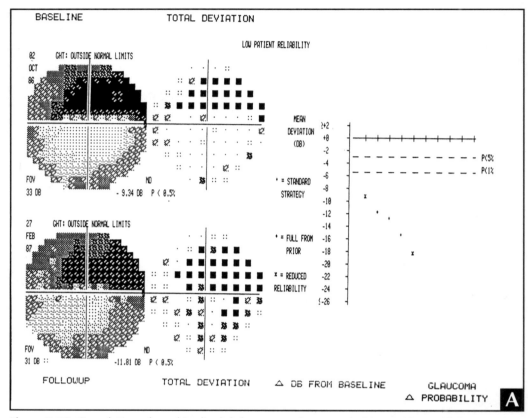

Figure 8-20. Completion of an altitudinal defect over a 6-year period in a patient with low-tension glaucoma and temporal arteritis. A. Baseline, B. Follow-up (Reprinted from Garber N. *Visual Field Examination.* Thorofare, NJ: SLACK, Inc; 1988).

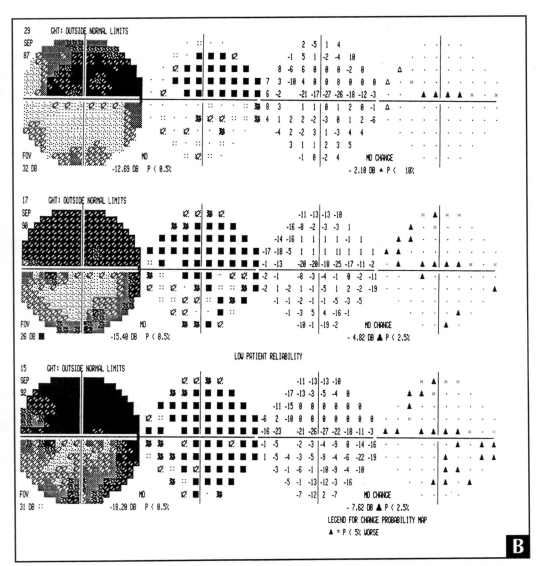

Figure 8-20 (B) Completion of an altitudinal defect over a 6-year period in a patient with low-tension glaucoma and temporal arteritis, continued (Reprinted from Garber N. *Visual Field Examination*. Thorofare, NJ: SLACK, Inc; 1988).

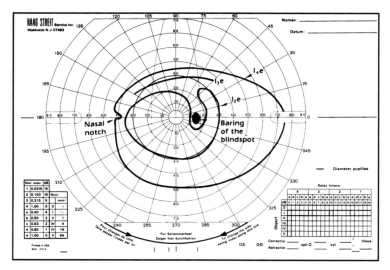

Figure 8-21. Glaucomatous field patterns showing baring of the blind spot and a nasal notch (Reprinted from Garber N. *Visual Field Examination.* Thorofare, NJ: SLACK, Inc; 1988).

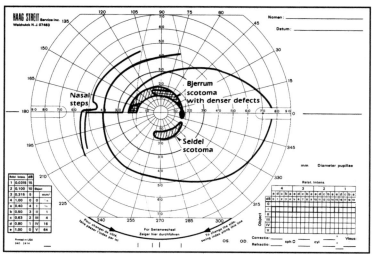

Figure 8-22. Nasal steps as seen in different isopters (Reprinted from Garber N. *Visual Field Examination.* Thorofare, NJ: SLACK, Inc; 1988).

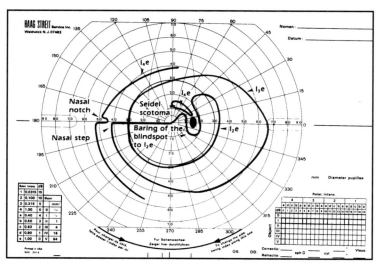

Figure 8-23. Common changes in the nasal isopters with glaucoma (Reprinted from Garber N. *Visual Field Examination.* Thorofare, NJ: SLACK, Inc; 1988).

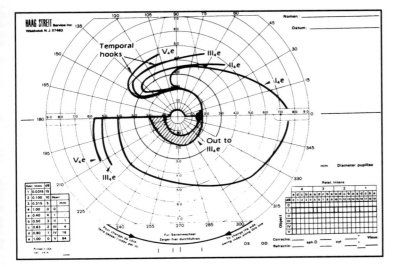

Figure 8-24. Progressive field changes with glaucoma showing contraction of the upper nasal isopters and a Bjerrum scotoma inferiorly (Reprinted from Garber N. *Visual Field Examination.* Thorofare, NJ: SLACK, Inc; 1988).

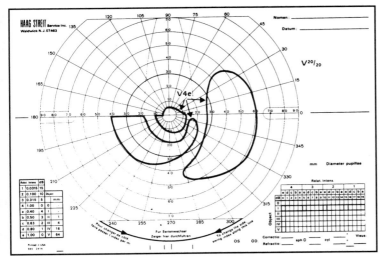

Figure 8-25. Severe field loss associated with glaucoma. Tunnel vision is present with sparing of the central field and good vision (Reprinted from Garber N. *Visual Field Examination.* Thorofare, NJ: SLACK, Inc; 1988).

Chapter 9

Visual Field Defects Due to Neurological Disease

KEY POINTS

- Many neurological diseases, such as multiple sclerosis, tumors, and strokes, may affect the visual pathways and lead to visual field defects.

- The pattern of the visual field loss may help to locate the site of the pathology within the central nervous system.

- Lesions occurring at or behind the optic chiasm cause visual field defects respecting the vertical midline, usually in each eye.

Introduction

Visual field testing may be an important component in the evaluation of patients with neurological disease affecting the visual system. Due to the anatomy of the visual pathways, the pattern of visual field loss may precisely pinpoint the location of the causative lesion, allowing the clinician to select the proper neurodiagnostic studies and appropriate referral for specialty care.

Optic Disc Based Field Loss

Diseases affecting the optic disc include glaucoma (discussed in Chapter 8); congenital abnormalities and structural defects such as drusen, colobomata, and pits (discussed in Chapter 10); inflammatory disease; tumors; and ischemic disorders. Visual field defects caused by optic disc disorders tend to localize to one side of the horizontal midline due to the arrangement of the retinal nerve fibers. Any or all of the defects illustrated in the earlier discussion of glaucoma may also be seen with any optic disc based disease.

Papilledema

Swelling of the optic disc caused by increased intracranial pressure is called papilledema. This may be due to a variety of causes, including brain tumors, meningitis, encephalitis, intracerebral bleeding, and subarachnoid hemorrhage. A common cause is a condition known as psuedotumor cerebri, in which the intracranial pressure becomes elevated for unknown reasons. Visual field defects from acute papilledema may include enlargement of the blind spot, as illustrated in Figure 9-1. If the swelling persists, other patterns of disc-based loss may become evident.

Anterior Ischemic Optic Neuropathy

This condition, abbreviated AION, results from a disruption of blood flow to the optic nerve. Disc-based visual field loss occurs, with the most frequent defect being an altitudinal hemianopia, as illustrated in Figure 9-2.

Optic Nerve Lesions

Optic Neuritis

Optic neuritis is a common inflammatory disease of the optic nerve with many different causes, including demyelinating diseases such as multiple sclerosis. Any type of visual field defect may be seen in patients with optic neuritis. Often during the acute episode the visual function is so severely affected that the visual field is not measurable. Figure 9-3 illustrates both visual fields approximately 7 weeks after an attack of retrobulbar neuritis, showing nasal loss in both eyes.

Figure 9-4 illustrates the visual field 2 years after an attack of optic neuritis. During the acute attack the vision had dropped to light perception only, and later recovered to 20/60. Note the residual defect is a diffuse loss of sensitivity (large negative mean deviation).

Compressive Optic Neuropathy

Compression of the optic nerve may result from tumors, trauma, and orbital inflammatory disease. Figure 9-5 is from a patient with an optic nerve meningioma, demonstrating peripheral constriction.

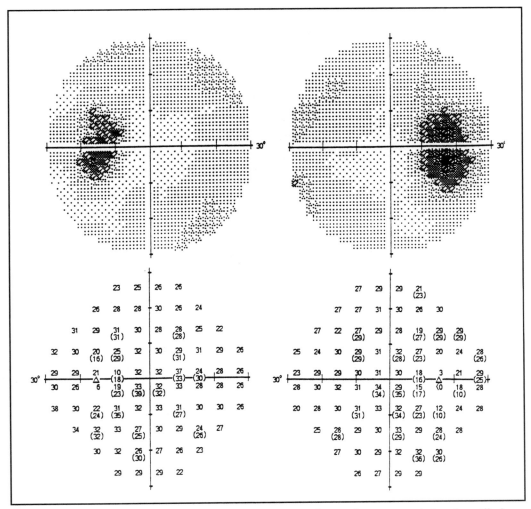

Figure 9-1. Threshold exam from both eyes of a patient with pseudotumor cerebri and papilledema demonstrating enlargement of the blind spot.

Figure 9-6 shows advanced loss due to optic nerve compression in a patient with Grave's disease, which may cause inflammation, swelling, and congestion within the orbit.

Optic Atrophy

The final result of many optic nerve disorders may be loss of the nerve fibers and atrophy of the nerve. The visual field from a patient with optic atrophy due to optic neuritis with final vision of 20/200 is illustrated in Figure 9-7. This field demonstrates diffuse loss of sensitivity and a central scotoma.

Chiasmal Syndromes

Recall that the optic chiasm is the anatomic point where optic nerve fibers from the nasal retina in each eye (serving the temporal visual field) cross to the opposite side. Figure 9-8 shows a typical bitemporal hemianopia resulting from damage to the chiasm following head trauma.

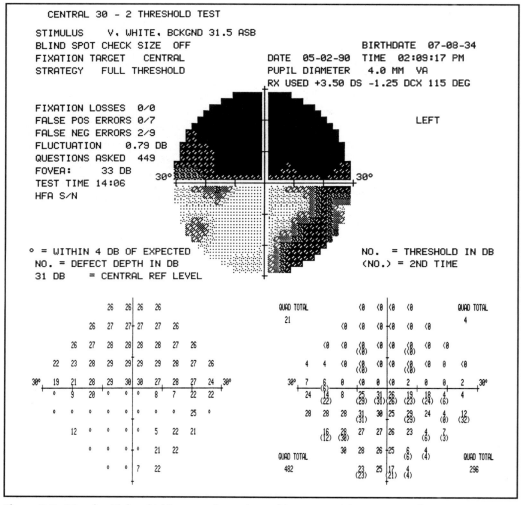

Figure 9-2. Stimulus V threshold exam of a patient with non-arteritic anterior ischemic optic neuropathy.

The pituitary gland lies just below the optic chiasm, and tumors of the gland often compress the chiasm, leading to visual field loss. Figure 9-9 is from a patient with a pituitary tumor, illustrating asymmetric bitemporal loss respecting the vertical midline in each eye.

Occasionally a lesion will affect a portion of the chiasm where one optic nerve enters. The resulting visual field defect, known as a junctional scotoma, will usually show marked loss in the eye with optic nerve involvement, and hemianopic loss in the other eye with involvement of the crossing nasal fibers. One such example is given in Figure 9-10.

Retrochiasmal Lesions

The visual pathways behind the chiasm carry information from the opposite side of visual space (ie, the left side of the brain receives the information from the right side of visual space and vice versa). Lesions affecting the retrochiasmal visual pathway produce homonymous visual field defects (on the opposite side), which become more congruous (symmetrical) the more posterior the lesion. Figure 9-11 is a congruous left homonymous hemianopia from a patient with a right parieto-occipital tumor.

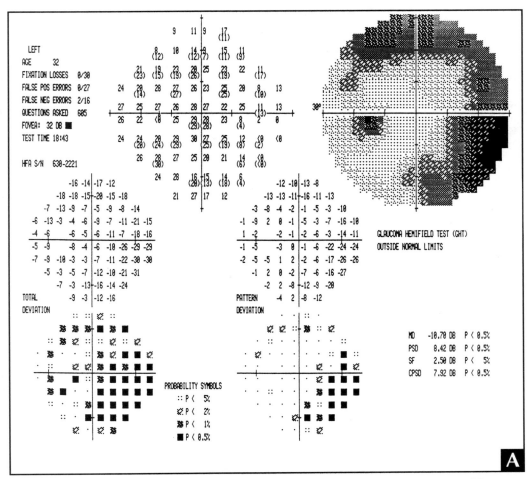

Figure 9-3. Threshold exam of left eye of a patient with optic neuritis demonstrating nasal loss in both eyes.

Figure 9-12 is a homonymous left superior quadrant hemianopia from a patient who had a right occipital lobe infarction.

Goldmann Fields in Common Neurological Disease

Swelling of the disc from papilledema or papillitis produces field loss by preventing light from reaching the peripapillary photorecptors, creating an apparent concentric enlargement of the blind spot as shown in Figure 9-13. This differs from the extension of the blind spot found in glaucoma where an "enlargement" of the blind spot occurs due to damage to nerve fiber bundles initially in the superior and inferior poles.

Bitemporal hemianopsias start as superior vertical steps, occurring occasionally in one eye only. As the damage increases, both eyes show temporal loss usually progressing towards fixation within the 30 degrees of eccentricity (Figure 9-14).

Temporal lobe lesions create field defects in the superior quadrant respect the vertical and are called "pie in the sky" defects. They are frequently incongruous (Figure 9-15)."

OphT

OphMT

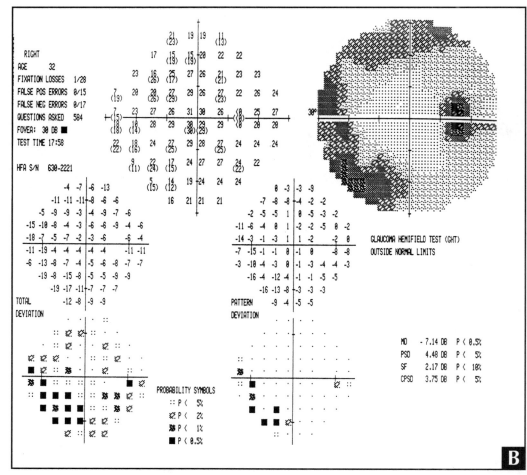

Figure 9-3 (B) Threshold exam of the right eye of the patient in Figure 9-3A.

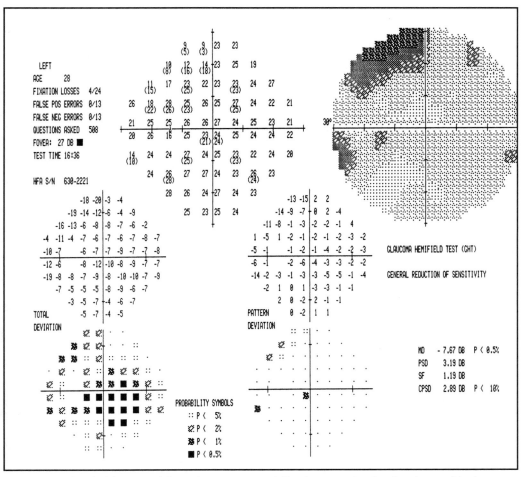

Figure 9-4. Threshold exam of the right eye 2 years following an episode of optic neuritis demonstrating residual diffuse loss of sensitivity.

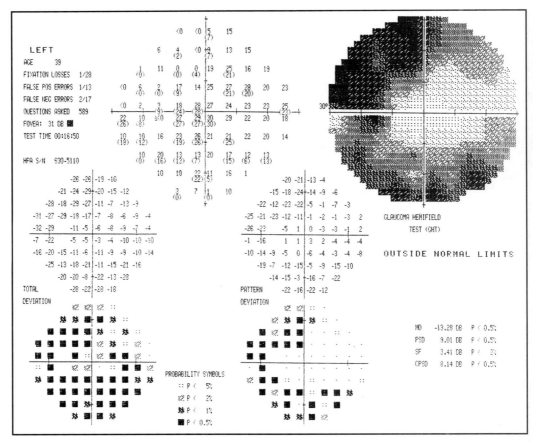

Figure 9-5. Threshold exam of the left eye from a patient with an optic nerve meningioma showing effects from optic nerve compression.

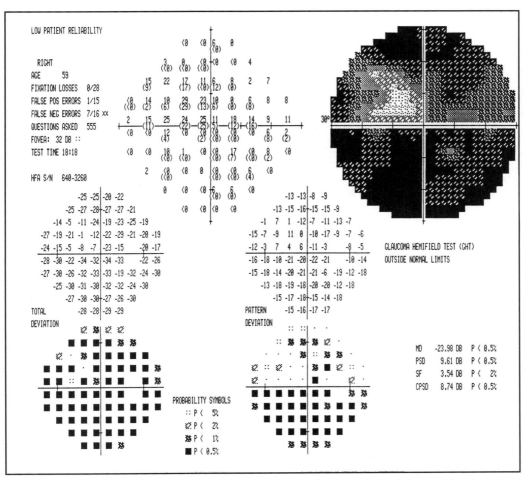

Figure 9-6. Threshold exam of a patient with optic neuropathy from Graves' disease also demonstrating the effect of optic nerve compression.

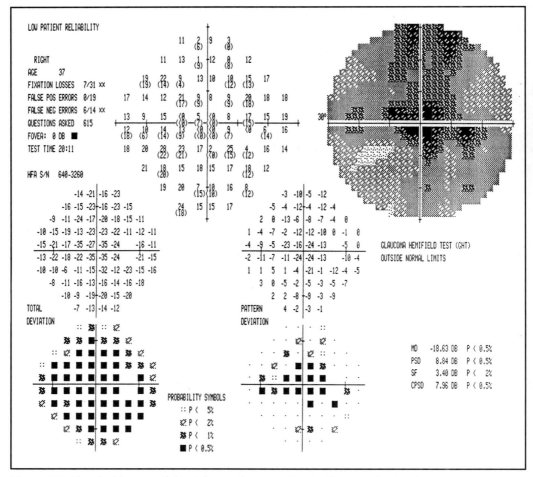

Figure 9-7. Threshold exam of the right eye from a patient with an optic atrophy.

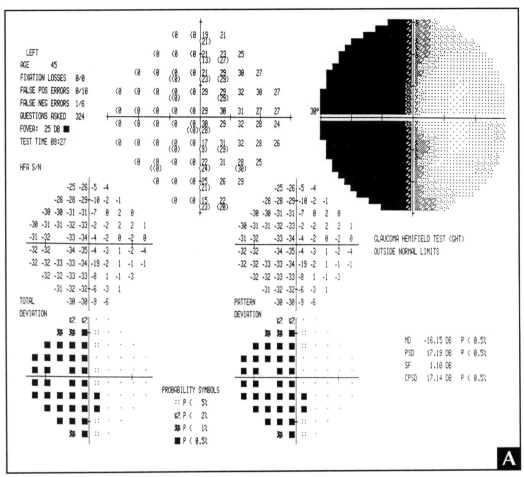

Figure 9-8. Bitemporal hemianopia in a patient 15 years following head trauma (left eye).

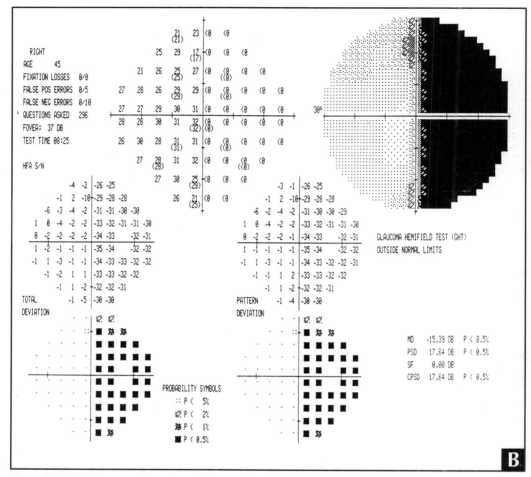

Figure 9-8 (B) Bitemporal hemianopia in a patient 15 years following head trauma (right eye).

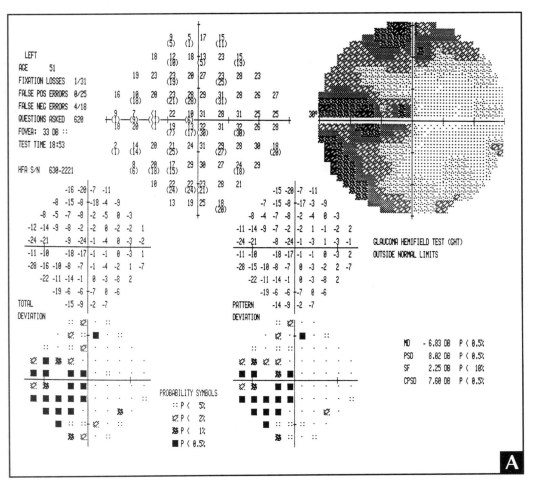

Figure 9-9. Threshold exam of left eye from a patient with a pituitary tumor, showing highly asymmetric bitemporal loss.

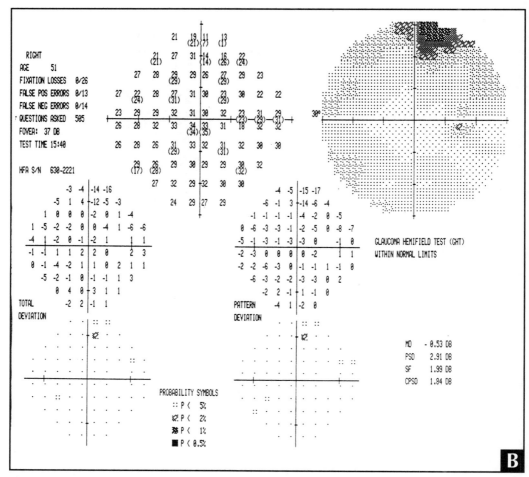

Figure 9-9 (B) Threshold exam of the right eye of the patient in Figure 9-9A.

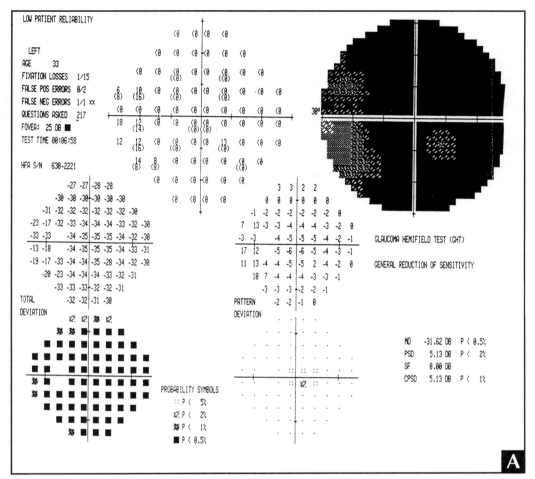

Figure 9-10. Threshold exam of left eye from another patient with a junctional scotoma from a pituitary tumor.

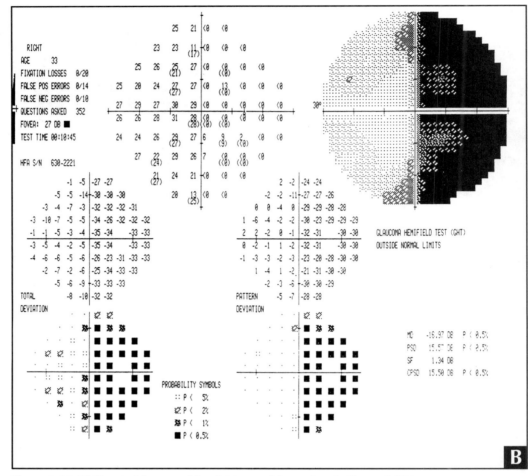

Figure 9-10 (B) Threshold exam of the right eye of the patient in Figure 9-10A.

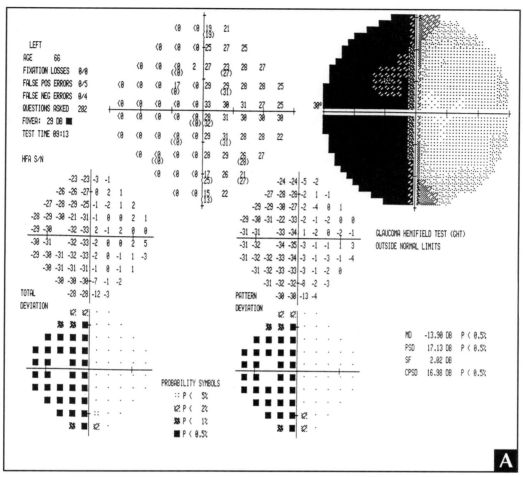

Figure 9-11. Complete left homonymous hemianopia from a parieto-occipital tumor (left eye).

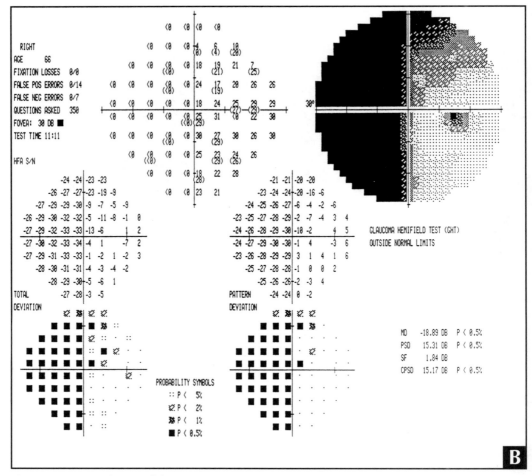

Figure 9-11 (B) Right eye of the patient in Figure 9-11A.

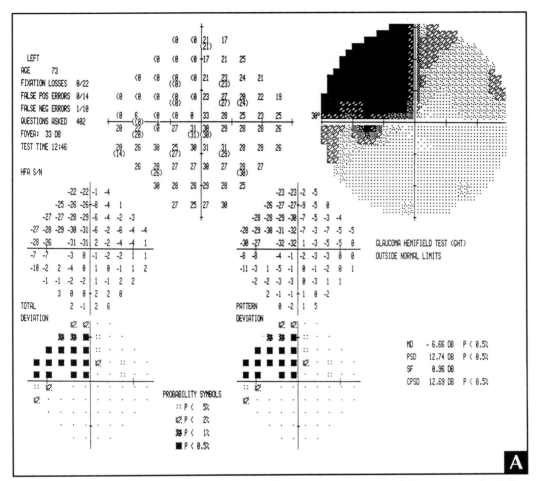

Figure 9-12. Left superior homonymous quadrant hemianopia in a patient following a stroke (left eye).

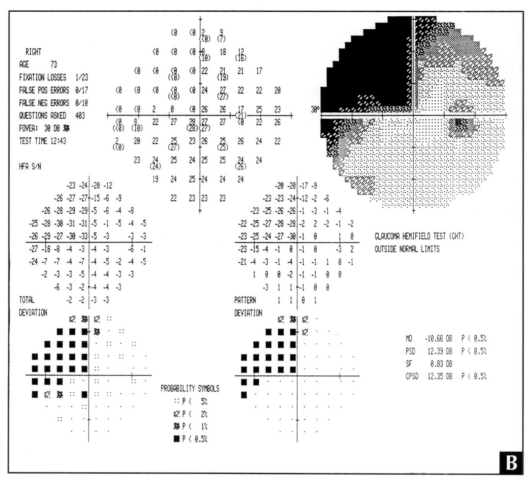

Figure 9-12 (B) Right eye of the patient in Figure 9-12A.

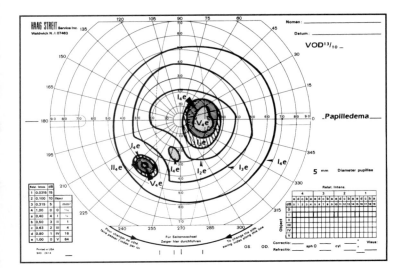

Figure 9-13. Visual field seen in papilledema (Reprinted from Garber N. *Visual Field Examination.* Thorofare, NJ: SLACK, Inc; 1988).

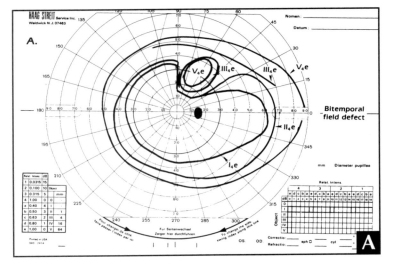

Figure 9-14. Field patterns seen when the pituitary gland compresses the chiasm where the nasal fibers cross (Reprinted from Garber N. *Visual Field Examination.* Thorofare, NJ: SLACK, Inc; 1988).

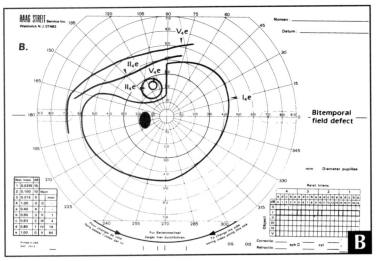

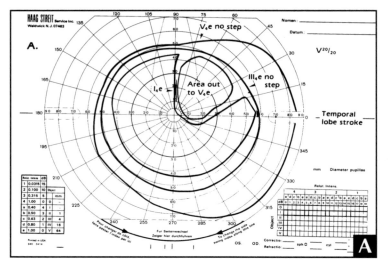

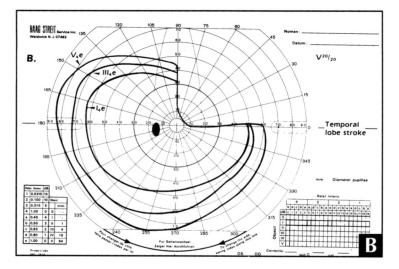

Figure 9-15. Field patterns seen in damage to the temporal lobe's optic radiations (Reprinted from Garber N. *Visual Field Examination*. Thorofare, NJ: SLACK, Inc; 1988).

Chapter 10

Visual Field Defects Due to Miscellaneous Conditions

KEY POINTS

- Visual field defects may be caused by structural abnormalities of the eye, media opacities, or retinal disease.

- Circulatory disturbances may present with visual field defects.

- Defects caused by various conditions may mimic those seen in glaucoma.

Defects Due to Structural Abnormalities of the Visual System

Enlargement of the Blind Spot

Because there are no photoreceptors on the surface of the optic nerve head, the area of the visual field containing the nerve head (15° temporally, straddling the horizontal midline) will appear as a "hole" in the visual field known as the physiologic blind spot. Enlargement of the blind spot due to papilledema was discussed in Chapter 9. Such enlargement may also result from a congenital abnormality of the optic nerve, or some variation of normal. Figure 10-1 shows the disc photograph and corresponding visual field of a congenitally aberrant optic nerve. There is a large scleral crescent, probably with exposed sclera visible, and multiple depressed points surrounding the center of the blind spot. The area of the probable blind spot has been circled.

Optic Pit

A structural defect in the temporal aspect of the optic nerve head may occur with the appearance of a localized excavation. One such typical optic pit and its corresponding visual field defect are shown in Figure 10-2. The visual field is typical of a nerve fiber bundle defect and could easily be confused with a glaucomatous defect.

Coloboma

Developmental abnormalities of the eye, in particular where the fetal fissure fails to close, frequently result in a defect in the inferotemporal aspect of the optic nerve known as a coloboma. Occasionally, structural defects will occur in the superior pole of the disc, resulting in inferior visual field defects. An example is shown in Figure 10-3. The remarkable aspect of this case is the symmetrical malformation of the superior poles of both optic nerves, and the similar inferior visual field defects.

Optic Nerve Drusen

Optic disc drusen are accumulations of a hyaline-like material within the optic disc anterior to the lamina cribrosa. Patients with disc drusen are usually asymptomatic, with normal visual acuity. Drusen are fairly common, and may occur in about 1% of the population. Optic disc drusen are usually discovered on routine ophthalmologic examination and may, if buried beneath the disc surface, cause elevation of the disc margin resembling papilledema. Sometimes the drusen will "erupt" or work their way to the surface of the nerve, causing a visual field defect. Figure 10-4 shows the visual field of a patient with optic disc drusen who had been observed as a glaucoma suspect because of the inferior nasal step.

 Defects Due to Retinal Disease

Macular Disease

The majority of patients with retinal disease do not require visual field testing because most of their disease is visible with the ophthalmoscope. The field in Figure 10-5 is from a 93-year-old with age-related macular degeneration. His foveal thresholds are reduced, right greater than left, and he has central depressions, right greater than left.

The visual field shown in Figure 10-6 is that of a patient with a macular hole. Even though the field was tested with the central fixation target, the defect and the blind spot appear to be shifted down because the

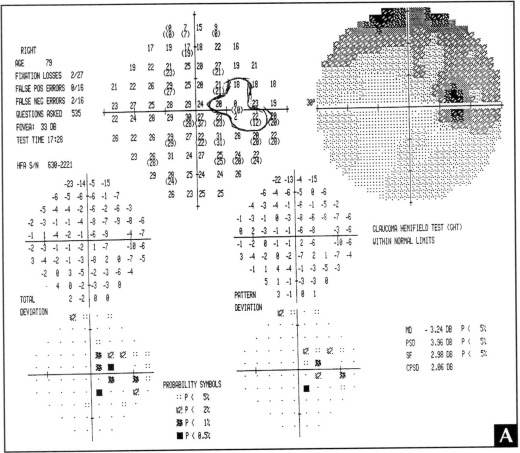

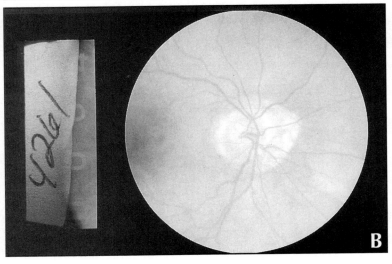

Figure 10-1. Disc photograph and visual field of a patient with a congenitally aberrant optic nerve, showing a scleral crescent and slight enlargement of the blind spot.

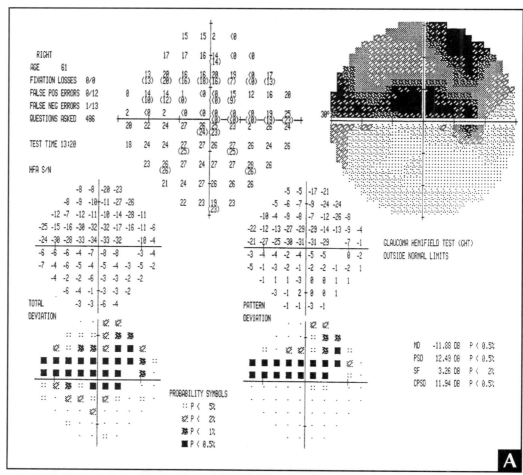

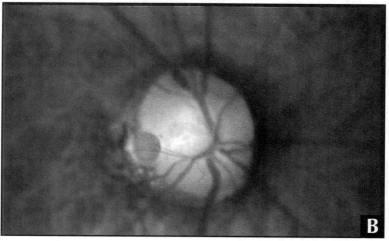

Figure 10-2. Disc photo and visual field of a patient with a congenital optic pit. The defect is a nerve fiber bundle defect.

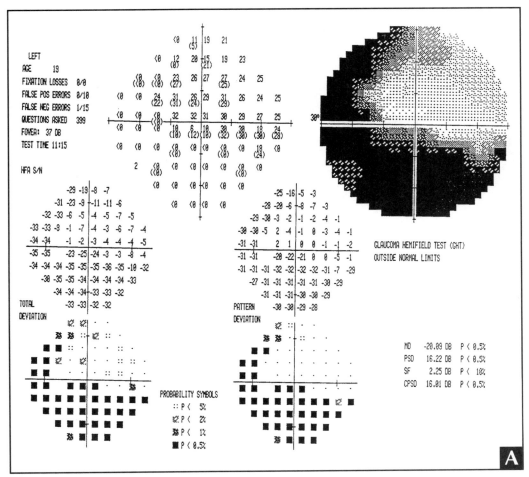

Figure 10-3. Visual fields (A and B) and disc photographs (C and D) of a patient with atypical colobomata of the optic nerve heads (left eye).

patient used his peripheral vision to fixate. Thus his eye was rotated during the test.

Retinal Detachment

Patients with retinal detachments rarely require field testing. The patient whose visual field is shown in Figure 10-7 underwent retinal detachment repair and complained of visual field loss. Although initially thought by a non-ophthalmologist to have redetached, clinical examination did not bear this out. A visual field was done because of his complaints. This loss pattern should never be confused with disc-based or neurological field loss because it does not respect either meridian. This patient did not have an acute process.

Retinal Dystrophies

Patients with retinal dystrophies often require visual field testing, either to document the extent of their loss for disability purposes or for diagnostic purposes when the diagnosis is not obvious ophthalmoscopically. Figures 10-8 and 10-9 are from patients with retinal dystrophies. The patient illustrated in Figure 10-8 has a rod-cone dystrophy. Both eyes demonstrate diffuse depression, and the left eye has a classic "ring"

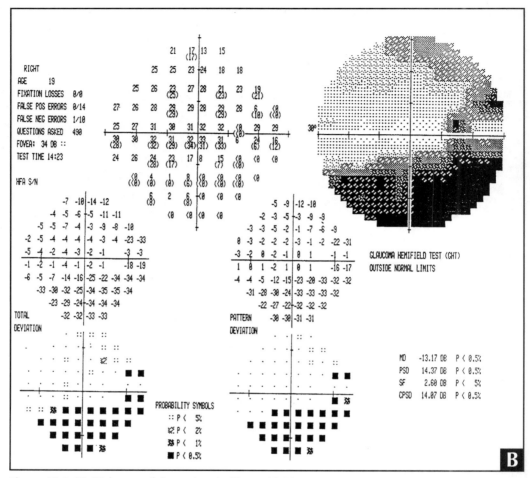

Figure 10-3 (B) Right eye of the patient in Figure 10-3A.

scotoma. The patient in Figure 10-9 has retinitis pigmentosa, with severe field loss, right much worse than left. Note the right eye required a stimulus V. The field was totally black to the stimulus III.

Retinal Scarring

Loss of vision following inflammatory disease in the visual system is related to destruction of tissue from the inflammatory process and replacement of tissue with scars. The visual field and disc photo shown in Figure 10-10 are from a patient with retinal scarring due to toxoplasmosis. The field defect is an inferior arcuate scotoma, due to the loss of a wedge of superotemporal nerve fibers.

Choroidal Rupture

Blunt trauma can cause significant intraocular injury, as is the case of the patient whose fundus photo and visual field are shown in Figure 10-11. The visual field defect corresponds to the inferonasal choroidal rupture and macular scarring. Because the paracentral defect and temporal wedge defect respect the horizontal, these could be mistaken for disc-based defects.

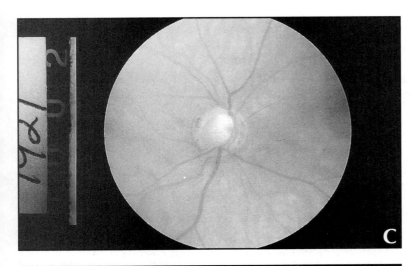

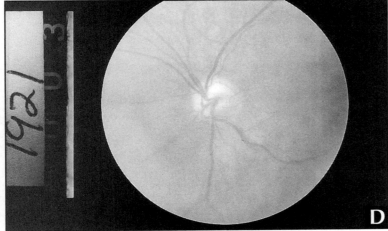

Presumed Vascular or Circulatory Problems (Systemic or Ocular)

The patient whose visual fields are shown in Figure 10-12 was under treatment for "low-tension" glaucoma. Each eye shows a disc-based superior nerve fiber bundle defect, and the optic nerves are both missing rim tissue at the inferior pole. These defects developed after the patient underwent uncomplicated coronary artery bypass grafting, and probably represent a form of "shock optic neuropathy." His ocular medications were discontinued and his IOP remained in the low to mid-teens, with no change in these visual fields over time.

Vascular accidents (strokes) would be expected to affect the visual field if a portion of the visual pathway was involved. The patient shown in Figure 10-13 had an occlusion of a cilioretinal artery. The resulting defect is therefore retinal based, rather than optic nerve based. It does, however, resemble the disc-based defects seen in glaucoma or mimicking syndromes (See Figure 10-12), and would be difficult to diagnose correctly without the proper history. The defect on the total deviation plot straddles the midline, as would be expected for a visual field defect due to a retinal lesion. There is also mild reduction in foveal threshold compatible with this artery occlusion.

Figure 10-14 is from a patient with background diabetic retinopathy who has undergone focal argon laser photocoagulation. The field shows a reduction in foveal threshold (20 dB), central loss, diffuse loss,

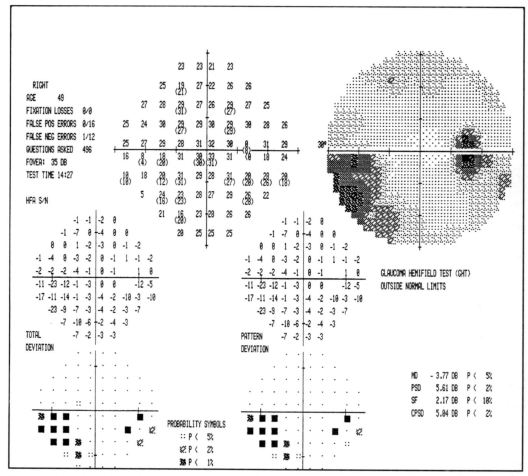

Figure 10-4. Visual field from a patient with optic nerve head drusen. The defect is a nasal step.

and some constriction. The central loss is attributable to diabetic macular edema.

The next two patients have a history of hypertensive crisis. The patient shown in Figure 10-15 complained of loss of vision in the center while retaining good visual acuity. The fields show bilateral central scotomata with relatively good foveal thresholds. The etiology of these defects is presumed to be an occipital lobe infarction.

Hypertensive crisis can occur as a complication of pregnancy, as experienced by the patient whose visual field is shown in Figure 10-16. She was not seen by an ophthalmologist during the acute episode, but rather weeks after the crisis. She complained of loss of peripheral vision from her left eye only, involving the lower left portion of her vision. The visual field loss detected on the 30-2 was only at the edge and could have been artifactual. Because of her insistence as to the extent of the loss, a peripheral 30/60 threshold test was performed, and the two printouts merged. The etiology of this defect is hard to pinpoint, but it is unilateral and therefore anterior to the chiasm, ie, optic nerve based. It most likely represents a segmental ischemic optic neuropathy.

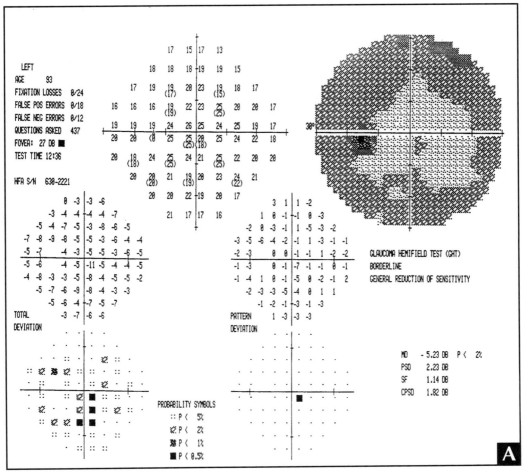

Figure 10-5. Visual fields from a patient with age-related macular degeneration. Note the reduction in foveal threshold and the central defects highlighted in the pattern deviation plots (left eye).

Media Opacities

Any opacity in the ocular media will reduce the amount of light reaching the retina. During a visual field test, the patient with a media opacity will demonstrate overall reduction in sensitivity values, because the stimuli will have to be made brighter than would otherwise be necessary. Cataract is the most common media opacity. Figure 10-17 shows a visual field typical of a patient with a cataract. Note the overall "darkening" of the graytone printout and the symbols in the total deviation probability plot, indicating that almost all of the points in the field are reduced in sensitivity. Figure 10-18 shows the series of visual fields from the same patient as in Figure 10-17. (Figure 10-17 is the third field from this series of five.) Note how the visual field shows overall darkening from the first examination as the cataract developed, followed by improvement after removal of the cataract between the third and fourth examinations.

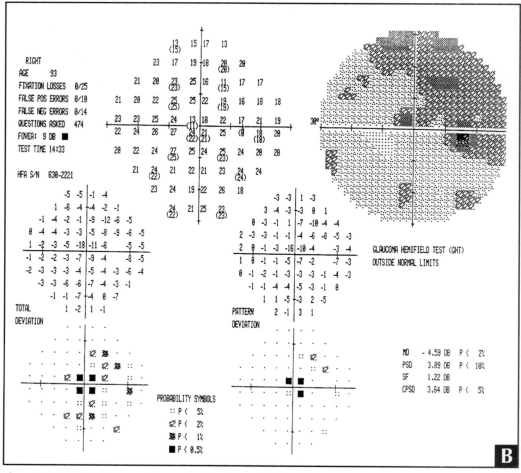

Figure 10-5 (B) Right eye of the patient in Figure 10-5A.

`OphT` Goldmann Fields

Drusen (German word for bumps) of the optic disc cause compression on the nerve fiber bundles in the nerve head. Field defects can produce progressive contractions, localized depressions, or scotomas. The most common field defects are inferior nasal contractions that curve toward the disc (Figure 10-19).

Retinitis pigmentosa produces diffused patterns of field loss starting where the rods are the densest at 30° to 60° eccentricities forming a ring of variable scotomas. These defects expand outward to the periphery and inward toward the fovea until blindness results (Figure 10-20).[1]

Reference

1. Garber N. *Visual Field Examination.* Thorofare, NJ: SLACK, Inc; 1988.

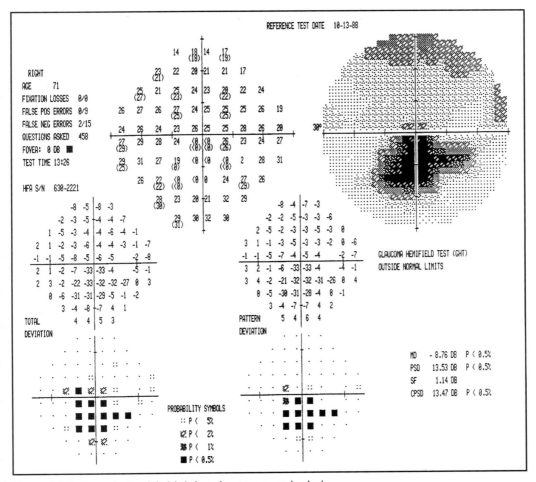

Figure 10-6. Central visual field defect due to a macular hole.

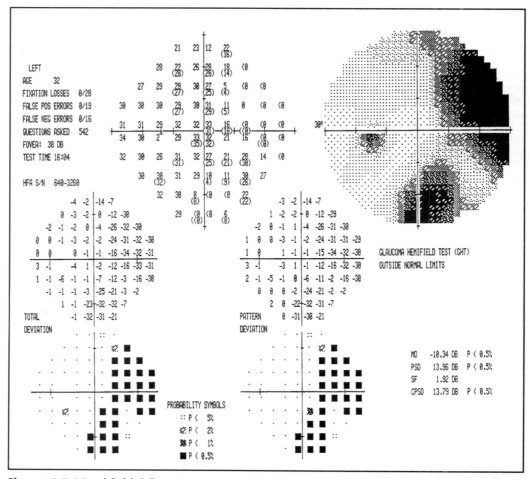

Figure 10-7. Visual field defects in a patient with a retinal detachment. Note that loss does not respect either meridian.

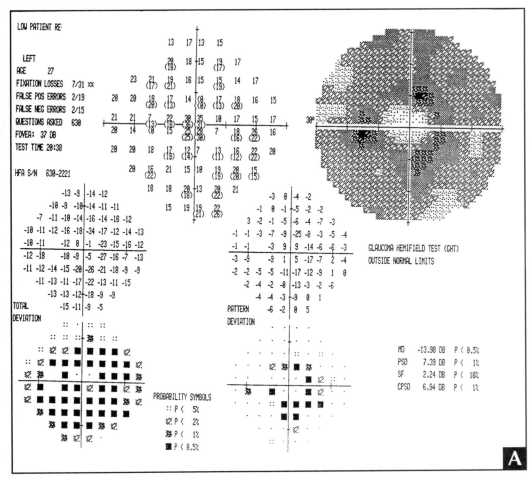

Figure 10-8. Visual field loss due to rod-cone dystrophy. Note the diffuse loss of sensitivity in each eye and the "ring" scotoma in the left eye.

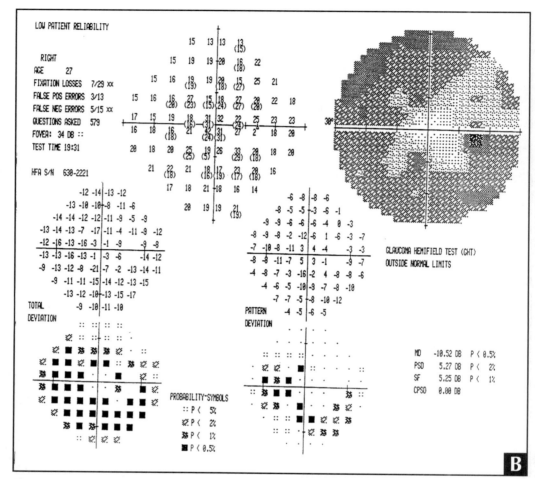

Figure 10-8 (B) Right eye of the patient in Figure 10-8A.

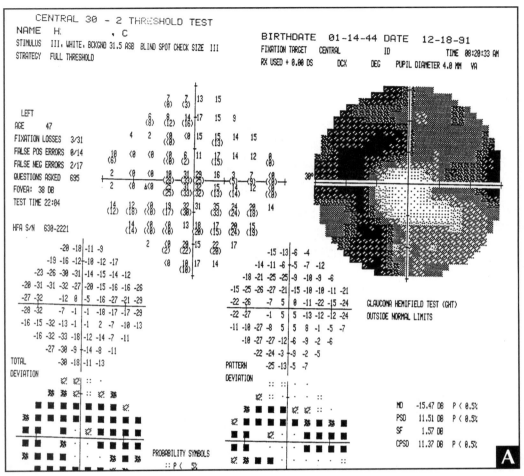

Figure 10-9. Visual field loss in a patient with retinitis pigmentosa (left eye).

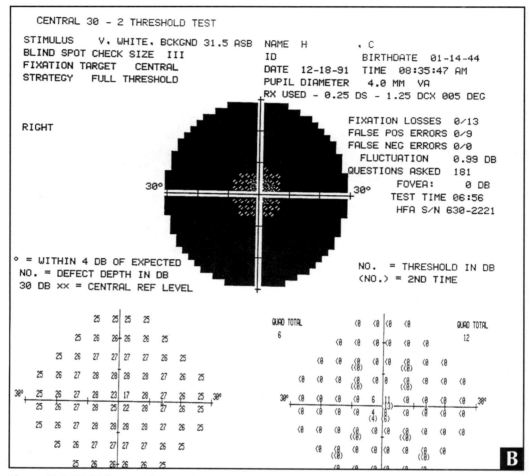

Figure 10-9 (B) Right eye of the patient in Figure 10-9A.

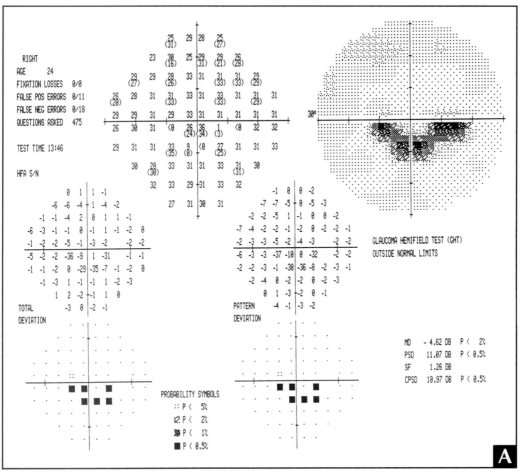

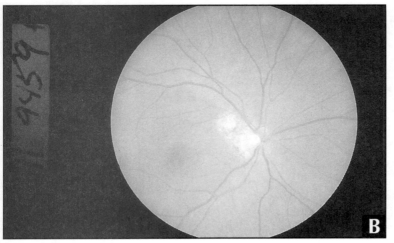

Figure 10-10. Visual field and fundus photograph from a patient with a retinal scar due to ocular toxoplasmosis.

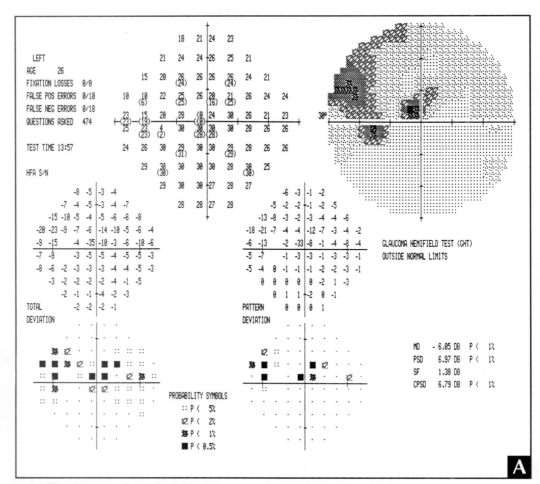

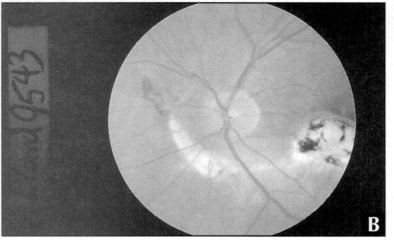

Figure 10-11. Fundus photograph and visual field following blunt trauma, with a choroidal rupture and macular scarring.

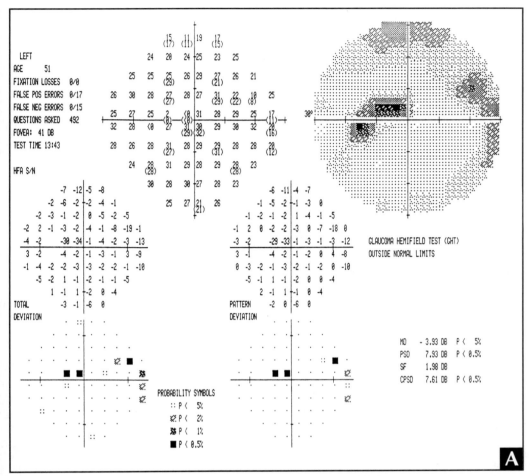

Figure 10-12. Bilateral nerve fiber bundle defects, which developed following open heart surgery, presumably due to "shock" (left eye).

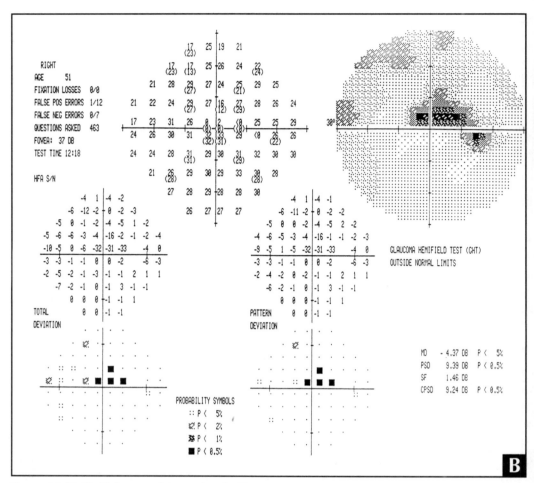

Figure 10-12 (B) Right eye of the patient in Figure 10-12A.

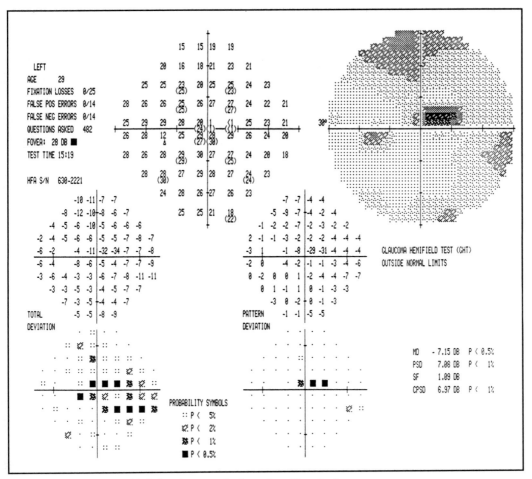

Figure 10-13. Visual field defect from occlusion of a cilioretinal artery.

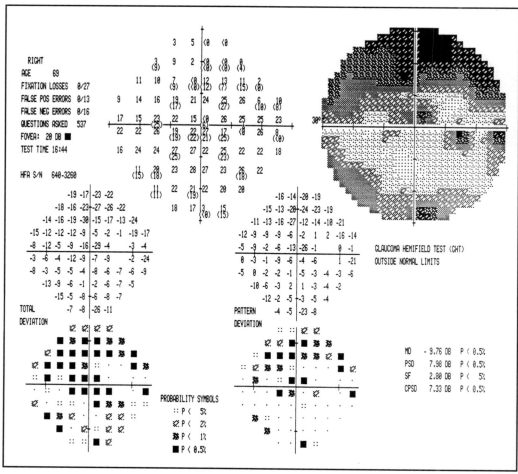

Figure 10-14. Visual field defects in a patient with background diabetic retinopathy.

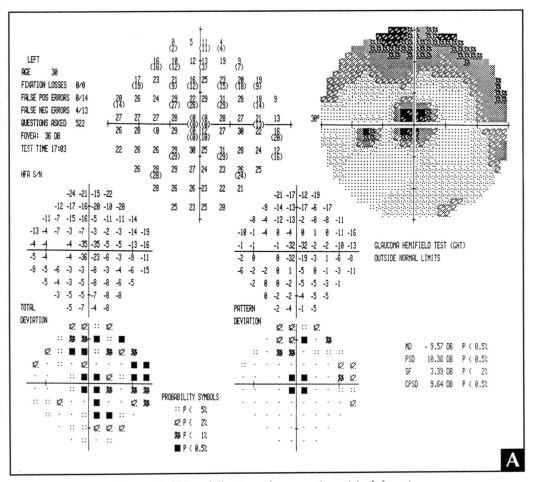

Figure 10-15. Central visual field loss following a hypertensive crisis (left eye).

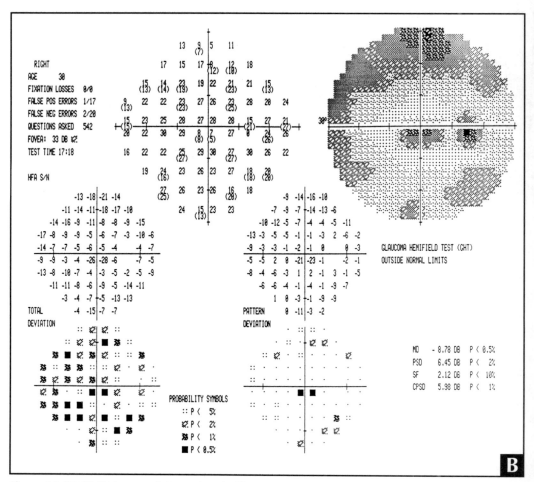

Figure 10-15 (B) Right eye of the patient in Figure 10-15A.

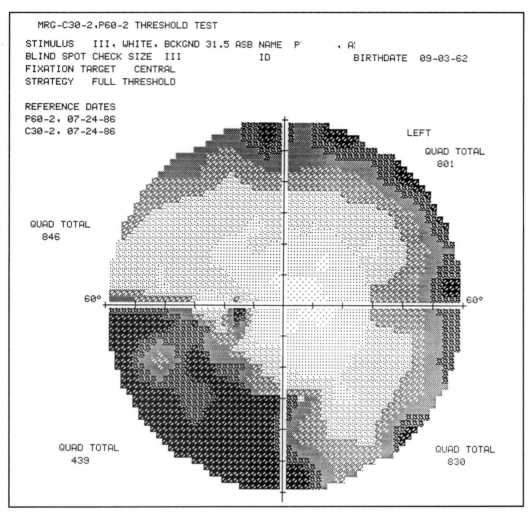

Figure 10-16. Peripheral visual field loss following a hypertensive crisis (merged 30-2 and peripheral 30/60, graytone printout).

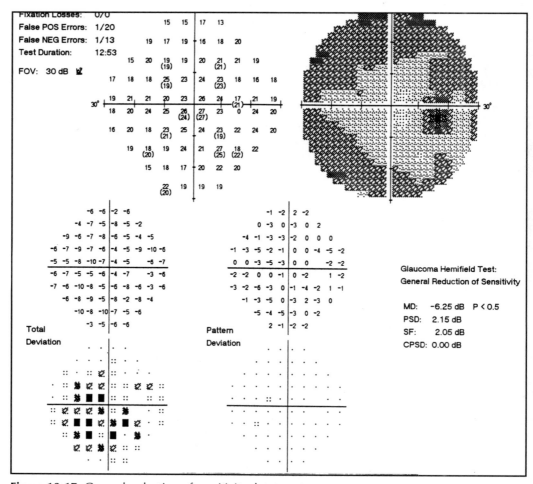

Figure 10-17. General reduction of sensitivity due to cataract.

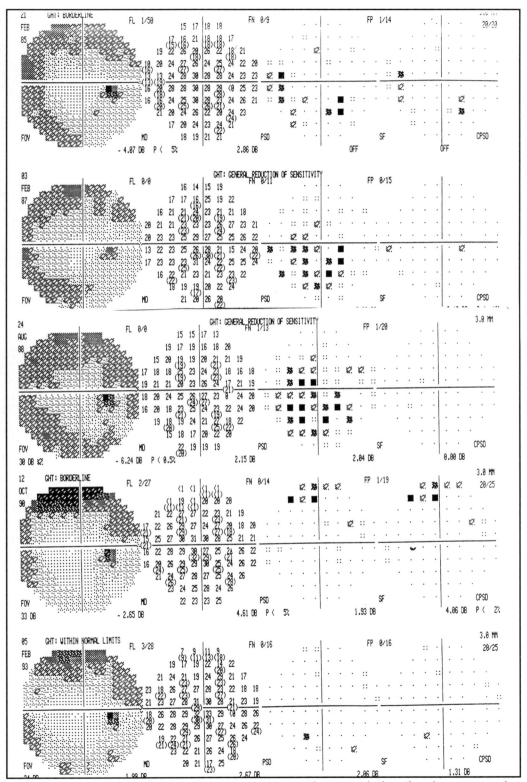

Figure 10-18. Visual field change over time in a patient with cataract before (first three tests) and after (last two tests) removal.

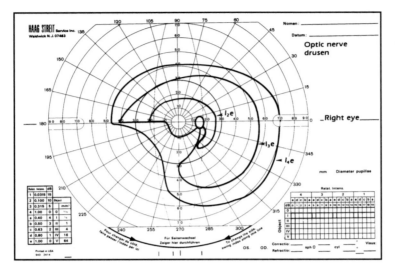

Figure 10-19. Optic nerve drusen causing field defects that mimic glaucoma. The defects may be progressive, and they tend to occur in the inferior nasal field first. Both eyes can be asymmetrically affected (Reprinted from Garber N. *Visual Field Examination.* Thorofare, NJ: SLACK, Inc; 1988).

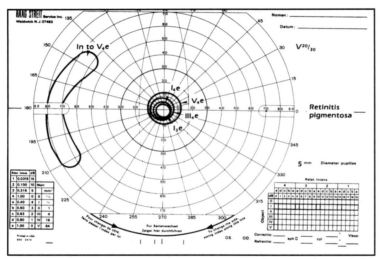

Figure 10-20. Field pattern in chronic, longstanding retinitis pigmentosa (Reprinted from Garber N. *Visual Field Examination.* Thorofare, NJ: SLACK, Inc; 1988).

Chapter 11

Advances in Visual Field Testing Equipment

KEY POINTS

- Visual field equipment and tests are constantly evolving.

- Semi-automated kinetic perimetry is highly interactive. Basically all the machine does is control the movement of the projector, open the shutter, record the patient responses, and plot the results.

- Kinetic fixation uses a moving fixation target. Stationary stimuli may then be used to test points simply by moving the fixation target.

- Gaze tracking uses corneal reflections to monitor eye movements during visual field testing.

- Short wavelength automated perimetry (SWAP) uses a yellow background and a violet test target. This stimulates the short-wavelength (blue) sensitive cones, which can be affected early in glaucoma.

- SWAP may be able to detect glaucomatous field loss up to 5 years before standard white-on-white perimetry.

Introduction

Visual field testing equipment has come a long way from the days of the tangent screen, when the invention of the Lumiwand™ was considered a big advance. Advances in electronics, computing power, information storage, miniaturization of components, and even in the concepts of what visual field testing is supposed to accomplish have all led to the development of new and more sophisticated testing equipment. New machines have expanded data storage capability using hard drives, optical discs, high capacity floppy disks, tape backup systems, gaze tracking systems, automated pupil diameter determination, and many other features. Not only has the hardware changed, but the test procedures themselves have changed to help us detect and follow the diseases that affect the visual field. This chapter presents some of the advances in perimeter design developed within the past 5 years.

Semi-Automated Kinetic Perimetry

Manual kinetic perimetry was discussed in detail in Chapters 3 and 4. Using a Goldmann perimeter, the perimetrist is responsible for controlling the placement and exposure of the stimulus, as well as recording the patient's responses and drawing the chart. The Humphrey Field Analyzer (with appropriate software) is now capable of performing a semi-automatic kinetic test. The process for this is detailed in the user's manual. Kinetic perimetry on the Humphrey perimeter requires a technician with the skills and knowledge required to perform Goldmann perimetry. This test modality is not automated in the same manner as threshold testing, and basically all the machine does is control the movement of the projector, open the shutter, record the patient responses, and plot the results (Figure 11-1). The test is highly interactive.

The test shown in Figure 11-1 was performed by a perimetrist who was unfamiliar with Goldmann testing. Only a single isopter was plotted, using the default I2e stimulus. The top of the figure shows what appears to be a vertical step. The blind spot was not mapped nor were static searches conducted for scotomata. The bottom of the figure shows the other printout option for kinetic tests, ie, a numerical printout listing each meridian tested, the starting and stopping point for the projector (degrees from fixation along that meridian for start and stop as well as the X,Y coordinates of the start and stop points), the isopter tested, the patient response, and the test type (standard or static).

A few key points are in order. First, the default stimulus is the I2e, and the machine does not do an automated determination of the suprathreshold stimulus intensity needed for the first isopter. However, the default can be changed, if desired. Second, the operator must select additional isopters to be tested, because they are not determined automatically. Up to 10 isopters can be plotted per eye. Scotomata can only be mapped if the operator pinpoints the starting location for the map. Central and paracentral scotomata can be searched for statically in custom scan mode by selecting the pad labeled "*static test currently off*" (it will then be turned on). The operator must then manually select each point to be tested statically, and that point will have a 1 second stimulus presentation. Any points not seen can then be explored as indicated above. Fixation behavior is not automatically monitored—the operator must watch the image of the eye on the video eye monitor. The image of the eye will move around the screen so as not to block out the moving target. Finally, printing can only be done on the internal dot matrix printer. If a laser printer is attached to the serial port, the machine will print the kinetic test on the dot matrix printer and then reset the system to the laser printer.

Multiple Stimulus Presentation Screening

The concept of rapidly screening the visual field by the simultaneous presentations of multiple stimuli was discussed in Chapter 5. The concept has been applied differently by at least two manufacturers of visual field testing equipment. The Dicon perimeter uses fixed light emitting diodes. The patient has a single

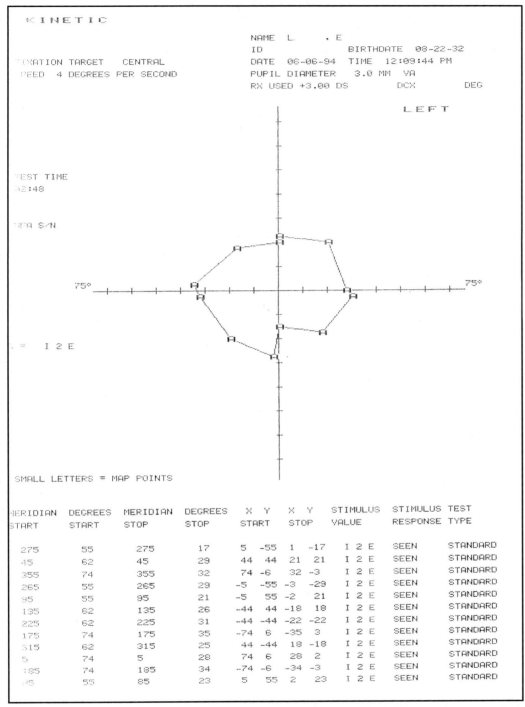

Figure 11-1. Top: single isopter kinetic field from the Humphrey Field Analyzer. Bottom: numerical printout from kinetic examination.

response button and pushes the button the number of times corresponding to the number of stimuli seen. Alternatively, the patient may indicate how many stimuli were seen by speaking the number into the microphone located just below the chin. Another automated perimeter on the market, distributed by Marco, uses four response buttons. The stimuli are presented one to a quadrant, and the response buttons correspond to the visual field quadrants. The patient then pushes the button for each stimulus seen. Theoretically, this technique could be used to rapidly perform threshold perimetry. The authors have no experience with this device.

Kinetic Fixation

All of the visual field techniques described so far require the patient to steadily fixate on a central (or fixed paracentral) target while stimuli are presented in the periphery of the field. This sort of "staring" is very fatiguing and difficult to maintain for prolonged periods of time. Dicon has incorporated a new method of fixation into the TKS brand perimeter series which uses a moving fixation target. This is known as kinetic fixation. The stimuli of these perimeters are 15 light emitting diodes (LEDs) at fixed locations within the bowl. Another target, attached by belts to translation motors, serves as the fixation device. The patient is instructed to follow the fixation light as it moves around the bowl and respond (verbally or with the response button) when lights are seen off to the side. The patient thus tracks the moving fixation target during the course of a test that may last 10 to 15 minutes; this is easier than trying to hold steady fixation on a stationary target.

In addition to possibly improving patient performance and acceptance of the test, kinetic fixation offers another benefit to perimeter design. Because the eye is moving, the position of the retina relative to a stimulus target is constantly changing. A single fixed stimulus could thus be used to test different portions of the visual field simply by varying the eye's position relative to the stimulus. The position of the eye is easily controlled by moving the fixation target. The need for a projector system to control stimulus presentations is eliminated, which in turn eliminates the motor and shutter noises that patients sometimes respond to. By using kinetic fixation and fixed LEDs, the Dicon perimeters are capable of testing any point in the visual field.

Gaze Tracking and Head Position Monitoring

The newest model from Humphrey Instruments, Inc, the Humphrey Field Analyzer II™ , has incorporated a gaze tracking device into its design. This device is capable of differentiating between head motion and deviations in location of the eye relative to the fixation target. When the patient is properly positioned in the machine for the start of an examination and the gaze tracking is initialized, the location of two small light reflections from the surface of the cornea is noted by the machine. Because of the corneal curvature, the distance between those reflections will change if the eye moves. The magnitude of the change is directly related to how much the eye has moved. Using this principle, the position of the eye at the time of each stimulus presentation is recorded and displayed on a continuous recorded strip (Figures 11-2 and 11-3).

The gaze tracking strip is located at the bottom of the printout. Each point on the horizontal line corresponds to a stimulus presentation, and each "spike" indicates the position of the eye relative to where it was at the time gaze tracking was initiated. The higher the spike, the more the fixation has deviated from its initial location. The field in Figure 11-2 illustrates good fixation behavior, with few large spikes and zero fixation losses recorded by the standard Heijl-Krakau method. The field in Figure 11-3, on the other hand, illustrates poor fixation behavior, with multiple large spikes and 19/28 recorded fixation losses.

The machine is capable of automatically making small movements of the chinrest to realign the patient if continuous misalignment is noted.

The new hardware design of the HFA II allows for some other sophisticated monitoring in addition to gaze tracking. The new head position monitor, or "vertex monitor," is capable of detecting if the patient's head has come off of the headrest, and will pause the test until corrective action is taken. This can help elim-

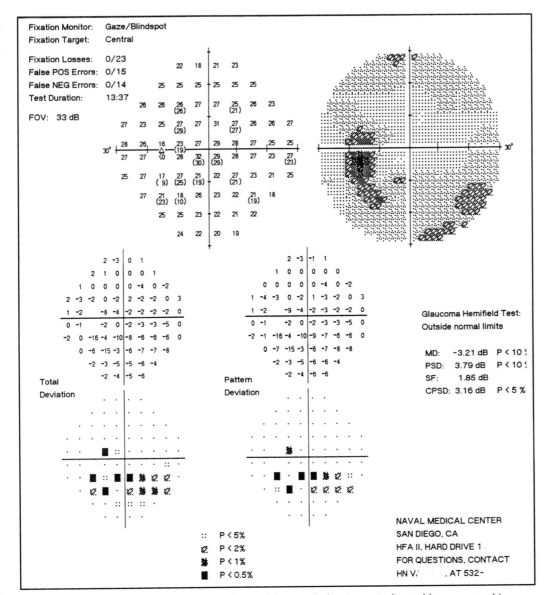

Figure 11-2. Visual field examination with good fixation behavior as indicated by gaze tracking.

inate lens artifacts. The machine is also capable of automatically determining pupil size and displaying it on the printout (not illustrated in these examples), expressed to 0.1 mm.

Short Wavelength Automated Perimetry (SWAP)[1]

Why a New Test Is Needed

The visual field examination remains the most important indicator of functional loss associated with glaucoma. However, standard automated achromatic perimetry (white flash on white background) may not

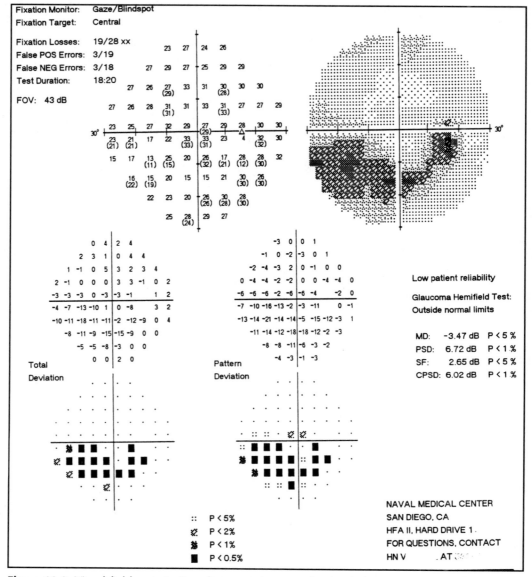

Figure 11-3. Visual field examination demonstrating poor fixation behavior on gaze tracking.

detect optic nerve damage at an early stage. Moreover, there can be considerable structural change in the optic nerve head in eyes with glaucoma before additional visual field loss is detected by standard achromatic perimetry. A new perimetric procedure, SWAP has been developed to address these problems.

The Rationale for SWAP

For several years, a loss of normal color vision has been known to be associated with glaucoma. Studies have indicated that blue-green color vision deficits are apparent early in the disease process. This region of color vision is handled by the short-wavelength cones and their neural connections. For an unknown reason, glaucoma either affects this system early in the disease process, or we are more able to detect early damage in this system. Evidence for blue-green deficits on central color vision tests, such as the Farnsworth-

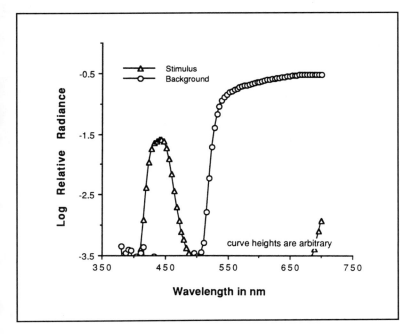

Figure 11-4. The log relative spectral radiance of the violet stimulus and yellow background used in SWAP in watts/steradian/m2 by nm. The x-axis spans the range of normal human vision from violet at 400 nm through blue, to blue-green, to green, to yellow, to orange, and red at 700 nm. These curves represent parameters recently agreed upon by several researchers who had each previously used different techniques for isolating the short wavelength mechanisms for visual field testing.

Munsell 100 hue test, the Farnsworth D-15, and the Pickford-Nicholson anomaloscope, is often present before peripheral visual field loss is found by standard perimetry.

However, color vision screening tests were not very useful for predicting the progress of the disease. Several factors other than glaucoma can affect these tests, such as lens density, pupil size, macular pigment, and other underlying medical diseases such as diabetes. Even when these factors are controlled and significant differences between normal eyes and eyes with primary open angle glaucoma can be documented, the separation between the groups is not sufficient for diagnosis and long-term management.

Two other factors that may have reduced the predictive ability of previous color vision testing in glaucoma were the emphasis on foveally-presented (fixated) stimuli and the use of tests originally designed to assess congenital color vision deficits. Tests which isolate short wavelength cone mechanisms, and which exploit the known loss of peripheral visual field sensitivity, are more appropriate for assessing eyes with primary open angle glaucoma. This is why SWAP was developed. By testing only the short wavelength sensitive mechanisms throughout the central 30° visual field, we are reducing any redundancy in the system, which may allow detection of the stimulus through some other visual pathway. This is unlike the stimulus in standard achromatic perimetry, which may be detected by any one of several systems.

What Is SWAP?

SWAP is a new technique that is identical to standard achromatic automated perimetry (white stimulus and white background) except that it tests only an isolated part of the color vision system, the short-wavelength (blue) sensitive cones, and their neural connections.

The key parameters necessary to isolate the short wavelength system are a broad-bandwidth bright yellow background of approximately 500 nm to 750 nm inside the perimeter bowl, and a Goldmann size V (1.8° visual angle, 64 mm²) violet test target centered at a wavelength of 440 nm (Figure 11-4).

The stimulus duration is 0.2 seconds. The yellow background adapts the rods and the middle wavelength and long wavelength-sensitive cones so they are much less able to detect the violet test stimulus. The color of the stimulus is centered in the wavelength range where the short wavelength cones can detect it best. With this set-up, an increase in stimulus intensity of approximately 15 dB is required before any other component of the visual system can detect the stimulus. All other aspects of the test are identical to standard perimetry.

How Useful Is SWAP for Diagnosis and Management of Glaucoma?

A series of results from two independent prospective longitudinal studies of SWAP have shown that the test is more sensitive for detecting early abnormalities than is standard achromatic automated perimetry. SWAP successfully differentiated between normal and glaucoma eyes. It showed deficits in ocular hypertensive and glaucoma suspect eyes up to 3 years prior to standard field loss, especially in eyes classified as high risk. The location of the short wavelength visual field defects was often the same as that later detected with standard visual field testing. Additionally, in glaucoma eyes, short wavelength fields have indicated more extensive damage across the retina than standard visual fields, and they have shown progressive loss sooner. SWAP also has similar test-retest reliability, short-term fluctuation, and long-term fluctuation as that of standard perimetry. Preliminary studies have also shown SWAP to be effective for diagnosis and follow-up of visual field loss associated with optic neuritis (Johnson CA, unpublished data) and with secondary and normal tension glaucomas. Indeed, it may be that SWAP might detect glaucomatous visual field loss up to 5 years before standard white-on-white perimetry.

With SWAP, both age and cataract can be taken into account and thresholds adjusted accordingly through the use of probability plots and statistical analyses such as the Glaucoma Hemifield Test. These analyses will be available on the Humphrey's internal statistics package when the normative database needed to perform them is completed.

The prospective longitudinal studies of SWAP are in their seventh year of following eyes with glaucoma and ocular hypertension. Additionally, SWAP has been included as an ancillary measure of visual function in a large multi-center study on the treatment of ocular hypertension sponsored by the National Eye Institute, National Institute of Health. Hence, SWAP is the only new diagnostic tool for glaucoma to have undergone this type of validation.

Adaptation of the Humphrey Visual Field Analyzer for Performance of SWAP

SWAP is now available on newer models of the Humphrey Visual Field Analyzer. Earlier models of the Field Analyzer can be modified with a kit which can be installed by the Humphrey service representative. This kit includes the necessary hardware and software modifications to perform the test. Once installed, the test is offered as an option to standard white-on-white testing for all screening, thresholding, special, and custom tests.

To access the SWAP version of a test, select the desired test (ie, 30-2, 24-2, *neurological*, etc) and the test eye as usual. When the test display screen appears, select *change parameters*. Highlight the *blue-yellow* option in the lower right corner of the screen and then select *return*. When the test screen reappears, the words *blue-yellow* should appear in the upper left corner of the display under the test eye. Continue the test as usual. When the test is completed *save to disk* as usual.

All print options will be available when the normative database is completed; however, the only accurate printing option currently available is in *numeric dB*. In the upper left corner of the printout, the test is designated as SWAP by the notation *stimulus V, blue, bckgnd yellow* and by the words *blue yellow* above the selected eye (Figure 11-5).

Reliability indices for fixation loss, false positive errors, false negative errors, and fluctuation are available on the printout. On rare occasions, testing the blind spot with a size V target is a problem, and the operator will need to either switch to a size III or turn the blind spot check off and self-monitor the fixation carefully.

At present, care should be taken when interpreting the results of SWAP fields. The test has only been

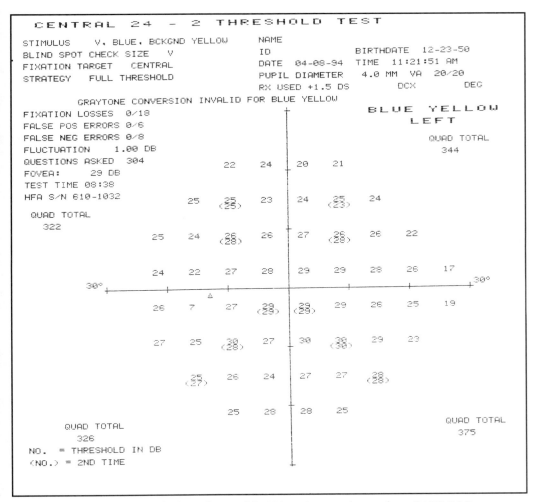

Figure 11-5. Visual field results from the modified Humphrey perimeter for a SWAP 24-2 program. Current printouts give reliability indices and threshold in numeric dB.

adequately evaluated for diagnosis and management of glaucoma using the 24-2 and 30-2 threshold tests. More research is needed to evaluate the effectiveness of the test for diagnosis and follow-up of other ocular and neurological disorders.

At the time of this printing, blue-yellow testing is available on some models of the Humphrey Field Analyzer and some Octopus™ perimeters from Interzeag, Inc. Age-matched normal controls are not available for SWAP data but should be available in the future.

Reference

1. Sample PA, Weinreb RN. Short wavelength automated perimetry. In: Choplin NT, Edwards RP. *Visual Field Testing with the Humphrey Field Analyzer.* Thorofare, NJ: SLACK Incorporated; 1995.

Chapter 12

Interpretive and Analytical Software for Automated Perimeters

KEY POINTS

- Interpretative software is only a tool for helping the eyecare provider identify abnormalities in the visual field examination. The software cannot readily differentiate artifactual loss from that due to any disease process.

- The final significance of the visual field test in the management of the patient, be it diagnosis or treatment, rests in the correlation of the visual field finding to the patient's clinical information.

- Major diagnostic or therapeutic decisions should not be made solely based on the visual field unless it makes sense. Nor should decisions be based on changes observed in a single examination, particularly where the test results may be subject to a certain amount of variability.

- The field examination should be carefully examined to make sure it was performed correctly (refractory, add, pupils, placement, etc), and repeated if any doubt exists.

Introduction

The printout from an automated perimeter is very different from the chart generated from a tangent screen exam or Goldmann perimetry. Interpretation of results requires an understanding of the principles of automated perimetry, particularly the concepts of attenuation (as measured by the decibel scale), threshold, and how threshold is determined. A thorough understanding of the island of vision analogy and how it is mapped is also essential. These concepts were discussed in Chapters 1 and 5.

When the Humphrey Field Analyzer was first introduced, the concept of normal threshold values was based on the "hill of vision" model. In other words, the visual field had an expected "shape" based upon Traquair's analogy, and any departure from that expected shape was considered abnormal. The defect depth printout as illustrated in Figure 5-26 and as part of Figure 5-28 shows the departures from "expected" normal based on the hill of vision model. This "shape" model makes it easy to spot scotomata, but it may be difficult to identify diffuse depression unless there is some sort of reference level given. The Octopus perimeters, on the other hand, used "age-corrected" normal values, ie, a population of "normal" subjects was tested and current results are compared to a group of similarly aged people. This "height" model makes the identification of diffuse loss easy (most points show defects), but focal loss may be difficult to identify. Thus, in order to interpret visual fields you need to know what the "normal" standard is for the machine and software you are using.

A basic approach to interpretation involves determining what test and strategy were used, evaluating measures of reliability (Chapter 5), and determining whether or not any artifactual defects are present. Then the field is assessed as to the presence of diffuse loss alone, focal loss alone (and its nature), or a combination of diffuse and focal loss. Because these determinations may be difficult, various computer software packages have been introduced to help in the analysis and interpretation of automated visual field results. Some of these packages reside within the operating software of the perimeter while others require an external computer. The remainder of this chapter will describe some of the packages currently available.

Statistical Analysis for the Humphrey Field Analyzer— STATPAC™

In the mid 1980s, Allergan-Humphrey introduced an optional statistical analysis package for the Humphrey Field Analyzer called STATPAC. Additions and modifications were made available in 1989 as another option called STATPAC II. These packages allow for the analysis of single visual fields with respect to a normal reference population, as well as for the analysis of a series of tests for changes over time. The package resides within the operating software for the field analyzer and no external computer is required.

The STATPAC programs are analytical only and do not change the way in which the testing procedures are carried out; only the output format and data analysis are changed by this software. STATPAC compares the patient's threshold results at a given location with the frequency of that same result (and location) in the normal population. For a specific patient value, the difference from the mean value in the normal reference population can be determined, as well as what percent of the time such a value would be expected to occur in the normal reference population. A low value (for example, showing a large difference from expected normal, expected to occur in the normal population less than 0.5% of the time) thus has a very high probability of being "abnormal."

STATPAC is designed for, and can only be used with, central threshold tests which include the 24-1, 24-2, 30-1, and 30-2, using stimulus size III and a white test object. It may not be used on averaged or merged fields. It can be used with stored tests as well as later ones, because the analytical package does not change the way the test is performed. The package can also be applied to tests performed with the "full from prior data" threshold strategy, but cannot be used with the "fast threshold" strategy. Data obtained using the FASTPAC thresholding strategy can be analyzed, but a mixture of normal strategy and FASTPAC fields cannot. Because STATPAC makes calculations with reference to a database of "normals" of the same age as the patient, it is essential that the patient's birth date be correctly entered.

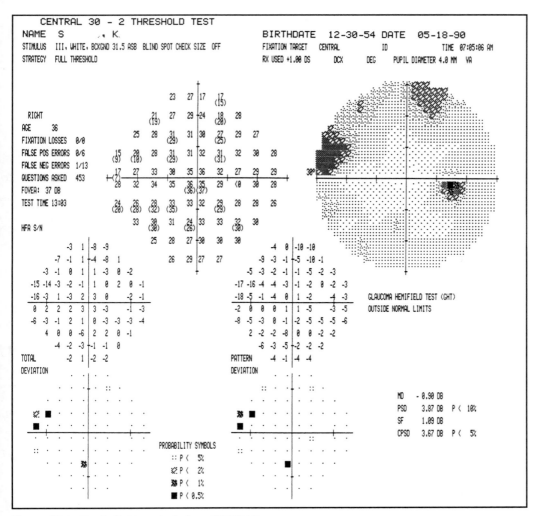

Figure 12-1. Single field analysis from STATPAC.

Analysis of a Single Visual Field

Figure 12-1 is an example of a STATPAC single field analysis. Patient identifying data and the test performed appear at the top of the page as before. The top grids are the usual patient measured threshold values (expressed in dB) and graytone formats, which are no different than those found on the standard Humphrey "triple" printout. The four bottom grids are the new analyses provided by STATPAC. Three types of analyses are provided for single fields—numerical deviation maps, probability maps, and global indices. STATPAC II adds a fourth—the glaucoma hemifield test.

The upper left grid displays the algebraic difference between the measured threshold values and the expected normal value for the patient's age for each test point, labeled "total deviation." In the grid just below, a symbol is assigned to each deviation value indicating the probability of finding such a deviation in the reference population. The darker the symbol, the greater the probability of abnormality, ie, that particular threshold value is seen less commonly among normal subjects. A key to the meaning of the symbols is given on the printout (not shown in Figure 12-1). In Figure 12-1, the nasal points showing threshold values of 12 dB (average of 17 and 7) and 15 dB (average of 20 and 10) would be expected to occur in less than 0.5% of the reference population (indicated by the black square symbols), ie, 99.5% of the age-matched nor-

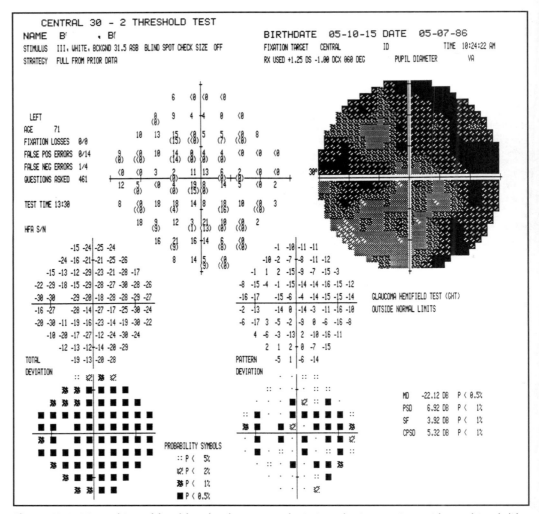

Figure 12-2. Unmasking of focal loss by the pattern deviation plot in a patient with combined diffuse loss from cataract and focal loss from glaucoma.

mals have higher threshold values at those points. Thus, those points are highly abnormal. The pattern is one of a nasal step.

Visual field loss, expressed in static perimetry as depressions of sensitivity, occur in two ways—diffuse (affecting the entire field, as might occur due to media opacities, incorrect refraction, or small pupils) and focal (scotomata). Diffuse loss, where all of the measured thresholds are below normal (or possibly above normal), can mask focal loss. STATPAC corrects the total deviation plot for diffuse loss, raising or lowering the overall height of the island of vision toward the mean for the reference population, and displays the results as the "pattern deviation" plot, printed on the right side of the page. Probability plots are displayed below the deviation plot. This process eliminates or diminishes general changes of height of the measured field, while focal loss remains clearly visible or enhanced.

Figure 12-2 is an example of a patient with a dense cataract and advanced glaucomatous damage. The adjustment from total deviation to pattern deviation reveals the nature of the focal loss, which is extensive in this case. Approximately 14 dB has been "added back" to the depressions noted on the total deviation plot. This "adjustment" is based on the distribution of the deviations noted in the total deviation plot. The "correcting factor" used to generate the pattern deviation plot is that value of deviation from the total deviation plot which lies at the 92nd percentile, with some consideration given for the location of each point as it is "corrected."

The four values given on the extreme right of the printout are the "global indices" (labeled MD, PSD, SF, and CPSD). These indices represent reductions in field data to single numbers and serve to summarize the field data. Probability (P) values are given for values outside of the normal range, indicating what percentage of the reference population may be expected to show the same or smaller value. The calculation of each index takes into consideration the location of each test point. Because the normal database contains the variance of each point around its mean value, these calculation methods allow deviations in the center of the field to be given more significance than equivalent deviations in the periphery (where the variance is greater).

The indices are:

1. Mean deviation (MD)—a measure of the overall height of the island of vision with regard to the reference population. A negative number indicates that the patient's island of vision lies below that of the reference population (ie, depressed). The mean deviation may represent many small depressions (overall depression) or significant loss in one part of the field and not in others.

2. Pattern standard deviation (PSD)—a measure of the shape of the island of vision. The normal island of vision has a smooth, regular contour that drops off from the center to the periphery in an expected way. The contour, or shape, of the island of vision is represented by the calculated value of pattern standard deviation. PSD estimates the non-uniform (ie, local) part of the deviation from normal, and may be thought of as the standard deviation of the numbers found in the total deviation array around the MD. If each point in the patient's visual field deviated from normal by the same amount (reflected in MD if different than zero), the PSD would be zero since the shape of that island of vision would parallel that of the reference population. If, however, a few points showed significant deviations, the spread of the deviations in the total deviation plot would be large, reflected in the PSD value. A large value indicates that the patient's island of vision does not have a smooth, regular contour; the larger the PSD, the more irregular the contour. Unlike MD, which is subject to diffuse effects, PSD is an indicator of scotomata within the field (assuming good patient reliability and low variability) regardless of the overall height of the island of vision. PSD may also be thought of as a measure of how each test point compares to its surrounding points; points that are depressed (ie, within scotomata) will have threshold values significantly different from neighboring points and give rise to a large PSD.

3. Short-term fluctuation (SF)—a measure of intra-test variability, specifically referring to the difference between repeated threshold measurement at points within one test session. It is calculated by measuring threshold twice at 10 predetermined points in the field (this is built into the Humphrey test software and is not unique to STATPAC) and then measuring the "spread" between the repeated measurements, averaging it over the field. In some older versions of the operating software SF must be turned on manually and is not automatically calculated, in which case STATPAC will print "off" instead of a number. Later versions of the software default to SF on. High values of SF may indicate unreliability of patient responses (which would be reflected in fixation losses, false positive responses, and false negative responses), or may represent increasing variability due to decreased sensitivity (either local or diffuse). Short-term fluctuation is one of the most important aspects of a static threshold perimetric test. It has been shown that increasing fluctuation in one area of the visual field is inversely related to the sensitivity of that area and may be predictive of impending loss.

   Figure 12-3 is an example of increased fluctuation preceding the development of a superior arcuate defect. The 10 points that are always double-determined are circled—note the large spread between repeated measurements in two points in the superior field (35 the first time, 25 the second, [indicated by parentheses], and 29 and 20), indicative of disturbance.

4. Corrected pattern standard deviation (CPSD)—PSD corrected for SF. As indicated above, the

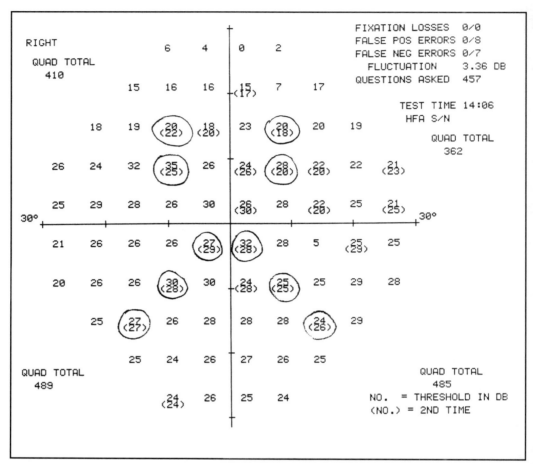

Figure 12-3. Fluctuation due to large spread in repeat measures of threshold in two points in the superior arcuate area. Points which are always double-determined as part of the SF test are circled.

PSD may be affected by high variability, ie, varying patient responses may make the contour of the island of vision appear irregular. STATPAC attempts to correct for this by factoring in the SF to the PSD and calculating the CPSD. If SF was not measured, STATPAC will print "off" instead of a number. This value thus represents the irregularity in the contour of the island of vision due to actual field loss, having removed the effects of patient variability. This number is thus the single most important indicator of the presence of scotomata within the field.

Visual field loss in glaucoma or optic nerve disease tends to occur in an asymmetric manner with respect to the horizontal meridian. Algorithms based on analysis of differences in clusters of mirror-image points across the horizontal meridian were developed during a natural history study of glaucoma. This has been termed the glaucoma hemifield test (GHT) and has been incorporated into STATPAC II.

Figure 12-4 shows how the test points are clustered into corresponding mirror-image areas above and below the horizontal axis. The differences in threshold for each cluster in the age-corrected reference population are determined and then compared to the mirror image cluster on the other side of the horizontal meridian.

A test that does not demonstrate significant asymmetry in departures from the reference population between the paired cluster points will be labeled as "within normal limits." Clearly asymmetric field defects

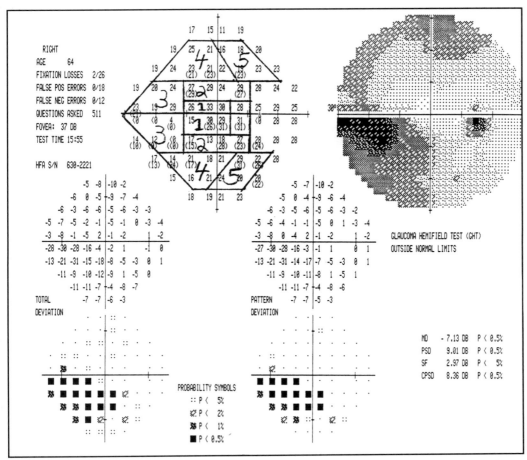

Figure 12-4. Clustering points into mirror-image groups above and below the horizontal meridian for the glaucoma hemifield test in STATPAC II.

will be identified as "outside normal limits" (Figure 12-5); shallow defects may be identified in this manner as well. "Borderline" results will be identified as such, and tests with abnormally high (Figure 12-6) or generalized reductions (Figure 12-7) in sensitivity can also be properly identified because the patient data has been compared to the age-corrected normals. Fields demonstrating abnormally high sensitivity should be looked at carefully for a high false positive response rate. Even though the field shown in Figure 12-6 met the criteria for reliability, there are multiple white scotomata and some impossible values in the field (55, 53, 47 40 dB). These are undoubtedly from false positive responses, but there were not enough catch trials for the rate to be abnormal. This patient had four out of 13 false positive responses; one more in the numerator or one less in the denominator and the rate would have met the 33% criteria to be indicated as unreliable.

The GHT will also report "outside normal limits" even if there is symmetrical loss across the horizontal, if the loss exceeds the 0.5% limit. The GHT has been shown to be comparable to other methods of cross-meridional analysis in terms of sensitivity and specificity for detecting glaucomatous loss. Figure 12-8 is an excellent example of how subtle inferior loss can be highlighted in a patient with early glaucoma. Note how the apparent superior temporal "defect" on the graytone falls within normal limits for STATPAC.

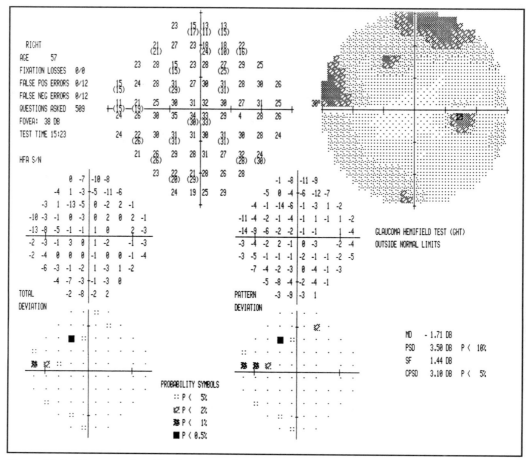

Figure 12-5. Glaucoma hemifield test outside normal limits.

Change in the Visual Field Over Time

A single visual field test is useful, and sometimes essential, for making or confirming a diagnosis. However, the management of a chronic disease such as glaucoma relies on determining the stability or deterioration of the visual field over time. In a test with significant variability in patient responses, sorting out true progression of defects from variability can be difficult. STATPAC and STATPAC II provide time analysis printouts designed to help in making this distinction. The later versions of the operating software will automatically locate all of the tests from a selected patient (for one eye), provided the patient's name has been entered the same way each time. If the patient has been tested with 30-2 and 24-2 tests, the time analyses will be displayed for the points common to both grids.

Rather than taking single field printouts and having to spread them over a desk or the floor to view them sequentially, STATPAC provides an overview printout (Figure 5-31), which can print the results of up to 16 tests on one page, displayed in chronological order. The printout contains the graytone, value table, total deviation probability plot, and pattern deviation probability plot for each test. Reliability and global indices are also displayed, and STATPAC II will print the results of the GHT across the top of each test. Results can be displayed for stimulus size III and V (Stimulus V overview). Scanning down the page allows for a rapid survey of the field changes over time. Figure 5-31 is an example of a worsening superior arcuate scotoma in a glaucoma patient.

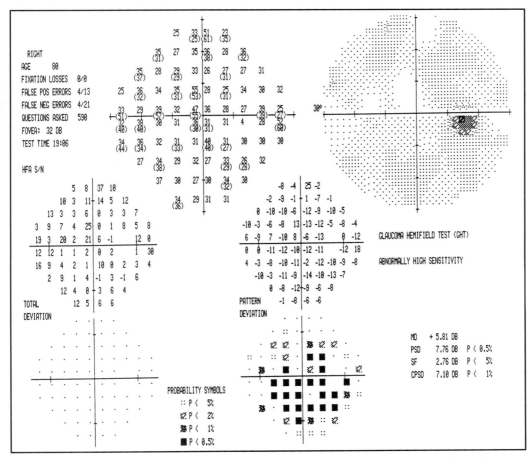

Figure 12-6. Abnormally high sensitivity indicated by the glaucoma hemifield test. Although the false positive catch trial rate was acceptable, there are a few points with "impossible" sensitivity. Mean deviations as high as that in this figure (+5.81) are usually due to false positive responses.

The overview printout is essentially raw data. The change analysis printout (Figure 5-32, same patient as Figure 5-31) provides an analytical summary of visual field results from earliest to most recent with up to 16 tests included. At the top of the printout is a modified histogram known as the box plot. This summarizes the total deviation plot by listing the differences between the patient's measured thresholds and the age corrected normals in order from the smallest to the largest. The scale on the left side of the plot lists possible departures from normal, ranging from greater than 10 dB above normal to more than 22 dB below normal. A "normal" box derived from the normal database is shown to the left of the scale. The patient's best value (smallest depression or largest positive departure from normal) corresponds to the 100th percentile and is represented by a horizontal bar at the top of the line. The worst value, or the largest departure from age-corrected normal, is the zero percentile and is represented by a horizontal bar at the bottom of the line. The top of the box represents the 85th percentile and the bottom represents the 15th. The median departure from normal (the 50th percentile) is represented by three horizontal bars inside the box. Interpretation of the box plot considers the overall length of the box, the location of the box relative to normal, the location of the median value, and the top and bottom end point lines. Diffuse depression without localized defects will result in a normally shaped box printed lower down on the scale. A scotoma comprised of only a few points will have a relatively normal box with a long negative tail. Worsening scotomata will result in elongation of the box over time, usually with the entire box "sinking."

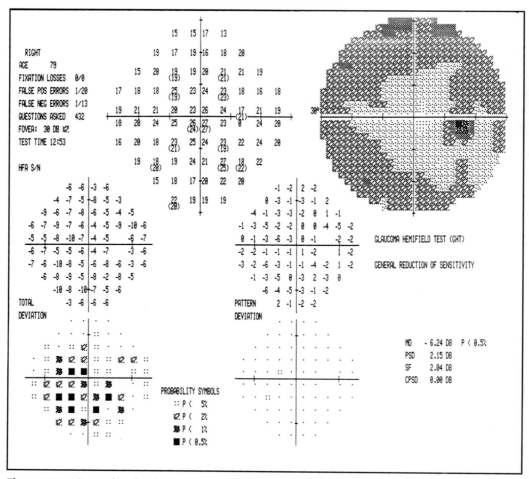

Figure 12-7. Generalized reduction in sensitivity identified by the glaucoma hemifield test.

In addition to the box plot, the change analysis printout contains a change summary of the global indices. Mean deviation, short-term fluctuation, pattern standard deviation, and corrected pattern standard deviation are plotted against time. The 5% and 1% limits for the reference population are represented by dashed lines. A patient value that falls below the 1% line, for example, would be expected in less than 1% of the reference population. A linear regression analysis on the mean deviation is performed if five or more tests have been conducted. The change in slope of the mean deviation over time (dB/year) is displayed, and a comment is made as to whether or not the change is statistically significant.

For observing glaucoma patients, STATPAC II adds a valuable time analysis printout known as the glaucoma change probability (Figure 5-33, same patient as Figures 5-31 and 5-32). It must be emphasized that this printout only applies to glaucoma patients (or suspects). Although the single field analysis will compare the patient to the standard age-corrected normal database, the glaucoma change probability compares the patient to a population of "clinically stable" glaucoma patients, not age-corrected normals. The analysis uses the patient's first two tests as baseline and subsequent tests as follow-up; if only two tests have been performed, it will use the first test as a baseline and the second test as a follow-up. If five or more tests have been performed, the first test will be ignored if the mean deviation falls significantly below the regression line of the subsequent tests (P < 5%) to account for learning effects. The analysis will not ignore unreliable tests; therefore a clinical judgment should be made to deselect tests that clearly showed the patient was inat-

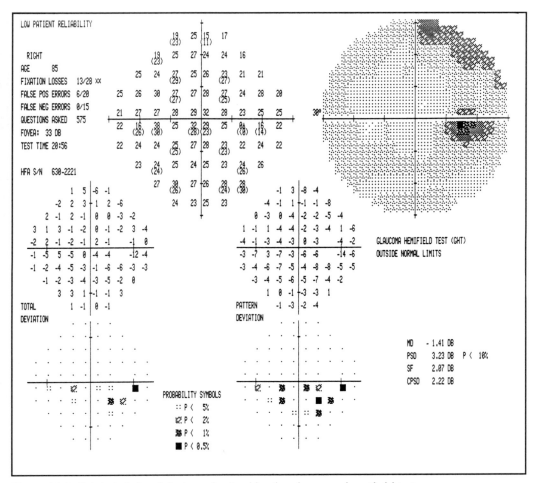

Figure 12-8. Subtle inferior defect emphasized by the glaucoma hemifield test.

tentive, inexperienced, or otherwise unreliable. The printout contains the graytone and total deviation probability plots for each test, and the results of the glaucoma hemifield test appear above the graytone. For each of up to 14 follow-up tests, a point-by-point age-corrected change from baseline (not the previous test nor the age-corrected normal thresholds) plot is provided. Positive numbers indicate improvement, negatives indicate worsening, and zero means no change. The fourth column under follow-up indicates the probability of the observed change (for each point) occurring in the population of stable glaucoma patients. An open triangle indicates that the observed improvement would be expected in less than 5%, and a black triangle indicates worsening observed in less than 5% of the stable glaucoma patients. Change in mean deviation is provided under the change from baseline plot with the probability of observing that change in the reference population. A modified linear regression analysis is performed on mean deviation and plotted at the top of the printout next to the baseline examinations. The glaucoma change probability analysis has been shown to be comparable to "traditional intuitive criteria" for identifying visual deterioration at individual points within a visual field. Figure 12-9 is another example of the glaucoma change probability plot, highlighting the areas of the visual field that deteriorated over time as the inferior nasal step developed in this patient with open angle glaucoma.

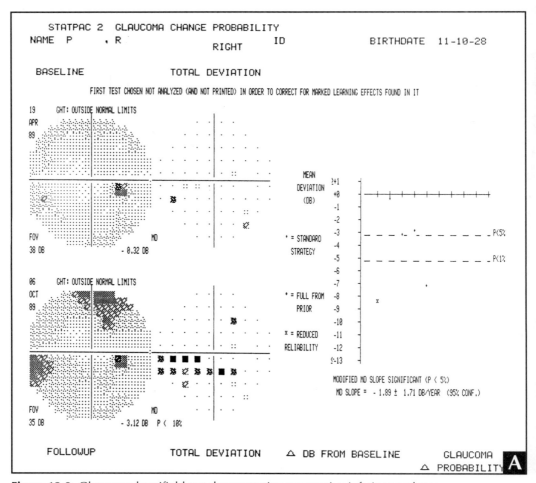

Figure 12-9. Glaucoma hemifield test demonstrating progressive inferior nasal step.

STATPAC for Windows

The video display of the Humphrey perimeter has limited capability for displaying visual field and data analysis results. Viewing multiple fields at one time is limited to printouts only, because multiple fields cannot be displayed on the machine. Data management, such as locating particular visual field results, is cumbersome due to the user interface, the need to scroll through disk contents one page at a time, and the relatively slow computer. STATPAC for Windows™ (SFW) is a software option offered by Humphrey Instruments, Inc that allows visual field data viewing and analysis using a DOS™-based IBM compatible personal computer running Microsoft Windows.

The SFW program is installed on the personal computer from floppy disks supplied with the package. Either a floppy disk drive is required in order to read data from the perimeter, or data must be transmitted to the computer through the perimeter's serial port. The program includes options for configuring the serial port of the computer to receive data from the perimeter. The Humphrey system uses proprietary floppy disk formatting. Visual field data stored on floppy disks normally cannot be read by a personal computer. In order to use field data from the perimeter with SFW, the data must be saved in a manner that will allow the SFW program to read it from the floppy disks. Therefore, the operating chips must be changed to make field data readable by the program. The chips are supplied with the SFW package. Once installed, a new pad appears

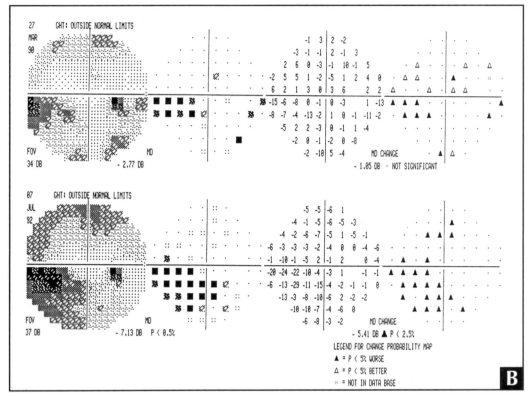

Figure 12-9 (B) Glaucoma hemifield test demonstrating progressive inferior nasal step, continued.

on the disk functions menu of the main menu which says, "*configure floppy disk for statpac for windows.*" This pad does not affect any data on the floppy disk except to make it readable by the SFW program. The data on the floppy disk must then be imported into SFW—the *import* button that appears on the button bar when SFW is opened will prompt for the insertion of a disk. The program then reads the disk and offers the option of selecting all files or individual files, using the computer's pointing device. All selected fields are then imported into one large file called "statpac.dat."

SFW is started as any Windows program would be. A blank screen appears with a menu bar (*file, records, charts, options*, and *help*) and a button bar (*import, open, print, right, left, prev, next, multi*, and *graph/num*). Selecting the *open* button displays a list of all patients on the hard drive—only data on the hard drive can be opened. Once a patient is selected, a list of the available visual fields is displayed. Clicking *OK* will open all of the fields for that patient, and up to six graytone images will be displayed on the screen, arranged chronologically from earliest to latest, left to right and top to bottom in a "graphic multi-tile raw threshold" chart. The *right/left* buttons toggle between right and left eye data. Both graphic and numeric multi-tile views are available, and each can be displayed as raw threshold, total deviation, pattern deviation, or global index views by selecting from the "chart" pull-down menu or by clicking the appropriate button. Multi-tile views cannot be printed. Individual fields can be selected for view by clicking on them, and any of the STATPAC printouts can be displayed on the screen, including the single field analysis, the three-in-one chart, the overview printout, the change analysis, and the glaucoma change probability. All of these charts can be printed. SFW does not print any double-determined thresholds, but rather prints the average of repeat measurements. One addition to the SFW printouts is a little box under the glaucoma hemifield test (on the right side of the printout beneath the graytone) with an indicator for the degree of abnormality. All of the change over time printouts have this little indicator for each field.

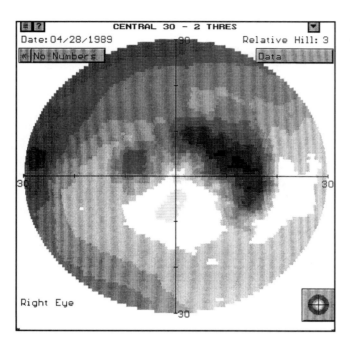

Figure 12-10. Grayscale printout from FieldView Omega from Dicon.

FieldView Omega™ from Vismed/Dicon

The Dicon TKS 4000 Autoperimeter, previously discussed, is an automated static threshold perimeter that contains limited data manipulation capability. FieldView™ software was developed to allow the retrieval of patient data from floppy disks into a personal computer and to offer alternative visual field data displays to the perimeter's internal printer. The current version of the software, Omega™, incorporates multiple display tools and age-related normal values for Dicon data. The software is also capable of reading Humphrey disks and displaying Humphrey visual fields in a variety of interesting ways. The software does not incorporate the age-related normal values for Humphrey data, and therefore analysis is limited to the hill of vision (shape) model. Age-corrected data is available for fields generated by the Dicon perimeter, and printouts may display the patient's results relative to the hill of vision model, the age corrected data, or both.

The FieldView Omega program runs under MS-DOS but does not use the Windows graphical interface. It does, however, allow display of multiple fields in their own windows which can be individually manipulated. When the program is loaded, a menu appears across the top with choices for fields (retrieve from hard disk or floppy), disk identification (label patient disk), displays (screen appearance), computer (setting perimeter options, printer set up, FieldView options, patient diskette formatting, and quit. Arranged vertically along the left side of the screen are various icons showing the options for displaying the data. They are, from top to bottom, numerical threshold values, grayscale, 3-D hill of vision, profile, ranked order, histogram, and isopters. A printer icon appears in the lower left-hand corner of the screen. The full screen or just one window can be printed.

An example of a grayscale printout from FieldView Omega is shown in Figure 12-10. The FieldView Omega software grayscale uses a 3 dB increment scale. Clicking the box just below the test date allows the raw threshold data to be superimposed on the grayscale (Figure 12-11). The 3-D hill of vision creates a three-dimensional view of the island of vision (Figure 12-12). The three-dimensional view can be rotated and tilted to allow multiple views. The isopter view (Figure 12-13) draws boundaries around the threshold data resembling a Goldmann field. The user can pick which isopter to display by dragging the small box in the scroll bar on the left of the window.

FieldView Omega allows the opening of up to four field windows. Each field can be displayed with the same or a different view. Figure 12-14 shows four visual fields over time from a glaucoma patient who developed a progressive superior arcuate scotoma over time.

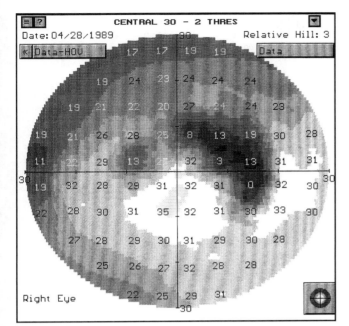

Figure 12-11. Grayscale with threshold data superimposed from FieldView Omega.

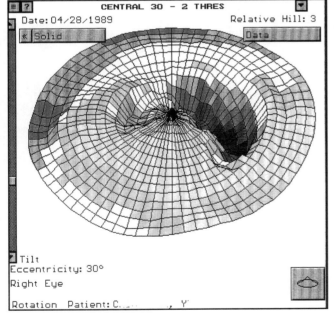

Figure 12-12. The three-dimensional hill of vision printout from FieldView Omega.

FieldView Omega can perform a "delta" analysis between any two fields (Figure 12-15). Points showing no change are indicated by a check mark, and a triangle symbol demonstrates points that are more than 5 dB below expected normal. Red triangles signify points more than 5 dB below normal in both tests, while green or blue triangles indicate points more than 5 dB below normal in only one of the tests, the color matching the background color of the test containing the abnormal value.

FieldView Omega can generate a number of reports. Figure 12-16 is an example of a Humphrey visual field as analyzed by the software. The printout contains the raw data (value table) and corresponding grayscale on the top, and the deviations from the expected hill of vision model displayed in a grid on the

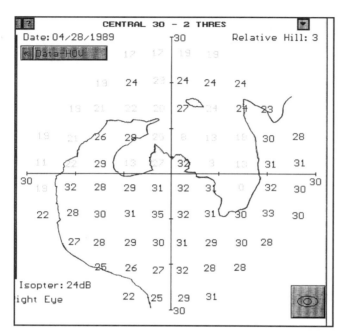

Figure 12-13. The isopter view from FieldView Omega.

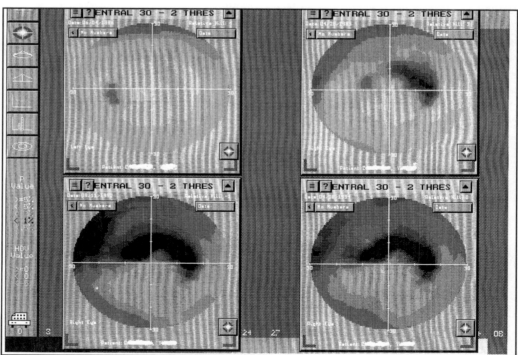

Figure 12-14. Multiple windows showing grayscales from four consecutive visual fields from the same patient from FieldView Omega.

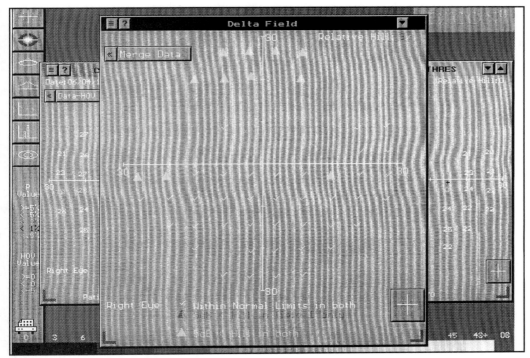

Figure 12-15. Full screen printout showing two visual fields and merge data delta field window from FieldView Omega.

lower left. A coded grid on the lower right displays the deviations by magnitude; the darker the symbol the larger the deviation. Similar printouts are available for tests performed by the Dicon perimeter and may contain similar graphical displays for differences from age corrected normals.

PeriData™ Visual Field Management Software

PeriData is a software package for IBM type personal computers from Interzeag, Inc, the company that manufactures and distributes the Octopus® line of automated perimeters. The software is designed to allow the viewing and analysis of visual field data from both the Octopus and Humphrey perimeters in a standardized format. The package contains a full library of statistical programs, has the ability to accept raw data from either perimeter, and can be used as an alternative to STATPAC. All familiar displays and printouts are available, and some other data presentation formats have been added, including color three-dimensional displays of the island of vision, cumulative defect curves (Bebie curve), stack bar analyses, graphical analyses of topographical trends (GATT), graphical analyses of numerical trends (GANT), and long-term overview trend analyses.

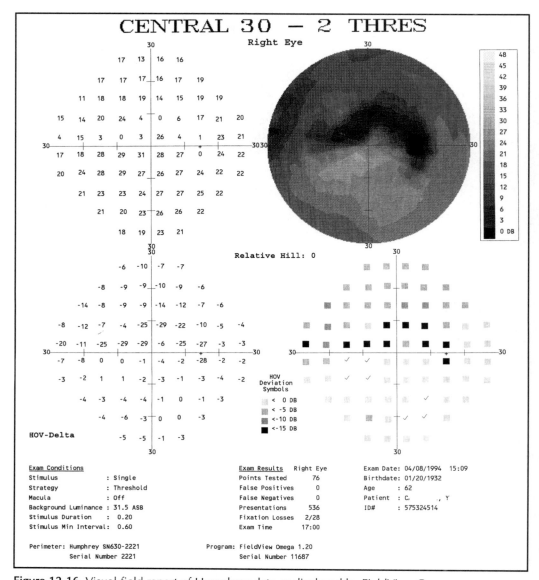

Figure 12-16. Visual field report of Humphrey data as displayed by FieldView Omega.

Bibliography

Adams AJ, Rodic R, Husted R, et al. Spectral sensitivity and color discrimination changes in glaucoma and glaucoma-suspect patients. *Invest Ophthalmol Vis Sci.* 1982; 23:516-524.

Allergan Humphrey. *STATPAC User's Guide.* San Leandro, Calif: 1987.

Anderson D. *Automated Static Perimetry.* St Louis, Mo: CV Mosby; 1992.

Asman P, Heijl A. Glaucoma hemifield test: automated visual field evaluation. *Arch Ophthalmol.* 1992;110:812-819.

Asman P, Heijl A. Evaluation of methods for automated hemifield analysis in perimetry. *Arch Ophthalmol.* 1992;110:820-826.

Bebie H, Fankhauser F, Spahr J. Static perimetry: accuracy and fluctuations. *Acta Ophthalmologica.* 1976;54:339-348.

Caprioli J. Automated perimetry in glaucoma. *Am J Ophthalmol.* 1991;111:235-239.

Caprioli J, Sears M, Miller JM. Patterns of early visual field loss in open-angle glaucoma. *Am J Ophthalmol.* 1987;103:512-517.

Choplin NT, Sherwood MB, Spaeth GL. The effect of stimulus size on the measured threshold values in automated perimetry. *Ophthalmology.* 1990;97(3):371-374.

Choplin NT. Technical advances in automated perimetry: statistical analysis of visual fields. *Ophthalmic Practice.* 1992;10(6):276-283.

Choplin NT. *Octopus Perimetry: A Meaningful Approach to Interpretation.* Huntington, WV: Cilco, Inc; 1985.

Choplin NT, Edwards RP. *Visual Field Testing with the Humphrey Field Analyzer.* Thorofare, NJ: SLACK Incorporated; 1995.

Drance SM, Anderson DR. *Automatic Perimetry in Glaucoma: A Practical Guide.* Orlando, Fla: Grune & Stratton Inc; 1985.

Drance SM. Diffuse visual field loss in open-angle glaucoma. *Ophthalmology.* 1991;98:1553-1538.

Duggan C, Sommer A, Auer C, Burkhard K. Automated differential threshold perimetry for detecting glaucomatous visual field loss. *Am J Ophthalmol.* 1985;100:420-423.

Garber N. *Visual Field Examination.* Thorofare, NJ: SLACK Incorporated; 1988 and 1991.

Haefliger IO, Flammer J. Fluctuation of the differential light threshold at the border of absolute scotomas: comparison between glaucomatous visual field defects and blind spots. *Ophthalmology.* 1991;98:1529-1532.

Haley MJ, ed. *The Field Analyzer Primer.* San Leandro, Calif: Allergan-Humphrey; 1987.

Hamill TR, Post RB, Johnson CA, et al. Correlation of color vision deficits and observable changes in the optic disc in a population of ocular hypertensives. *Arch Ophthalmol.* 1984; 102:1637-1639.

Harrington DO. *The Visual Fields.* 4th ed. St Louis, Mo: CV Mosby; 1976.

Heijl A, Lindgren G, Olsson J. A package for the statistical analysis of visual fields. In: *Seventh International Visual Field Symposium.* Amsterdam, Netherlands: 1986:153-168.

Herse PR. Factors influencing normal perimetric thresholds obtained using the Humphrey Field Analyzer. *Invest Ophthalmol Vis Sci.* 1992;33:611-617.

Heuer DK, Anderson DR, Feuer WJ, et al. The influence of decreased retinal illumination on automated perimetric threshold measurements. *Am J Ophthalmol.* 1989;108:643-650.

Holmin C, Krakau CET. Variability of glaucomatous visual field defects in computerized perimetry. *Albrecht v Graefes Arch Clin Exp Ophthalmol.* 1979;201:235-250.

Johnson CA, Adams AJ, Casson EJ, et al. Blue-on-yellow perimetry can predict the development of glaucomatous visual field loss. *Arch Ophthalmol.* 1993; 111:645-650.

Johnson CA, Adams AJ, Casson EJ, et al. Progression of early glaucomatous visual field loss for blue-on-yellow and standard white-on-white automated perimetry. *Arch Ophthalmol.* 1993; 111:651-656.

Katz J, Sommer A. Asymmetry and variation in the normal hill of vision. *Arch Ophthalmol.* 1986;104:65-68.

Katz J, Sommer A, Gaasterland D, Anderson D. Comparison of analytic algorithms for detecting glaucomatous visual field loss. *Arch Ophthalmol.* 1991; 109:1684-1689.

Katz J, Sommer A. Reliability indexes of automated perimetric tests. *Arch Ophthalmol.* 1988;106:1252-1254.

Lam BL, Alward WLM, Kolder HE. Effect of cataract on automated perimetry. *Ophthalmology.* 1991;98:1066-1070.

Lieberman MF, Drake MV. *Computerized Perimetry: A Simplified Guide.* Thorofare, NJ: SLACK Incorporated; 1992.

Lindenmuth KA, Skuta GL, Rabbani R, et al. Effects of pupillary constriction on automated perimetry in normal eyes. *Ophthalmology.* 1989;96:1298-1301.

Morgan R, Feuer W, Anderson D. Statpac II glaucoma change probability. *Arch Ophthalmol.* 1991;109:1690-1692.

Sample PA, Weinreb RN, Boynton RM. Acquired dyschromatopsia in glaucoma. *Surv Ophthalmol.* 1986;31:54-64.

Sample PA, Taylor JD, Martinez G, et al. Short-wavelength color visual fields in glaucoma suspects at risk. *Am J Ophthalmol.* 1993;115:225-233.

Sample PA, Weinreb RN, Boynton RM. Isolating the color vision loss of primary open angle glaucoma. *Am J Ophthalmol.* 1988;106:686-691.

Sample PA, Martinez GA, Weinreb RN. Color visual fields: a 5 year prospective study in eyes with primary open angle glaucoma. *Perimetry Update 1991/1992: Proceedings of the Xth International Perimetric Society Meeting.* Amsterdam, Netherlands: Kugler & Ghedini; 1993;473-476.

Sample PA, Weinreb RN. Progressive color visual field loss in eyes with primary open angle glaucoma. *Invest Ophthalmol Vis Sci.* 1992; 33:2068-2071.

Sample PA, Weinreb RN. Color perimetry for assessment of primary open angle glaucoma. *Invest Ophthalmol Vis Sci.* 1990;31:1869-1875.

Sample PA, Weinreb RN, Boynton RM. Blue-on-yellow color perimetry. *Invest Ophthalmol Vis Sci* (Suppl ARVO abstract). 1986; I 27 :159.

Sample PA, Weinreb RN. Variability and sensitivity of short-wavelength color visual fields in normal and glaucoma eyes. *Digest of Topical Meeting on Noninvasive Assessment of the Visual System.* Washington, DC; Optical Society of America; 1993:292-295.

Sample PA, Juang PSC, Weinreb RN. Short-wavelength automated perimetry for analysis of secondary and normal tension glaucoma. *Invest Ophthalmol Vis Sci* (Suppl, ARVO abstract). 1994;35:2189.

Sanabria O, Feuer WJ, Anderson DR. Pseudo-loss of fixation in automated perimetry. *Ophthalmology.* 1991;98:76-78.

Sommer A, Enger C, Witt K. Screening for glaucomatous field loss with automated threshold perimetry. *Am J Ophthalmol.* 1987;103:681-684.

Walsh TJ, ed. *Visual Fields: Examination and Interpretation.* San Francisco, Calif: American Academy of Ophthalmology; 1990.

Werner EB, Adelson A, Krupin T. Effect of patient experience on the results of automated perimetry in clinically stable glaucoma patients. *Ophthalmology.* 1988;95:764-767.

Werner E, Drance S. Early visual field disturbances in glaucoma. *Arch Ophthalmol.* 1977;95:1173-1175.

Werner EB, Saheb N, Thomas D. Variability of static visual threshold responses in patients with elevated IOPs. *Arch Ophthalmol.* 1982;100:1627-1631.

Whalen WR, Spaeth GL. *Computerized Visual Fields: What They are and How to Use Them.* Thorofare, NJ: SLACK Incorporated; 1985.

Zalta AH. Lens rim artifact in automated threshold perimetry. *Ophthalmology.* 1989;96:1302-1311.

Index